	DATE DUE		

When did I begin?

When did I begin?

Conception of the human individual in history, philosophy and science

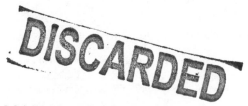

NORMAN M. FORD, S.D.B.
President of the Melbourne College of Divinity, Melbourne, Australia

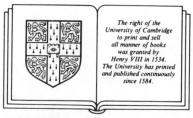

The right of the
University of Cambridge
to print and sell
all manner of books
was granted by
Henry VIII in 1534.
The University has printed
and published continuously
since 1584.

CAMBRIDGE UNIVERSITY PRESS

Cambridge

New York   Port Chester

Melbourne   Sydney

Published by the Press Syndicate of the University of Cambridge
The Pitt Building, Trumpington Street, Cambridge CB2 1RP
40 West 20th Street, New York, NY 10011–4211, USA
10 Stamford Road, Oakleigh, Victoria 3166, Australia

© Cambridge University Press 1988

First published 1988
Reprinted with minor corrections 1989
First paperback edition 1991

Printed in Great Britain at the University Press, Cambridge

British Library of Congress cataloguing in publication data
Ford, Norman M.
When did I begin: conception of the human individual in history, philosophy
and science.
1. Man. Conception. Philosophical perspectives
I. Title
128′.5

Library of Congress cataloguing in publication data
Ford, Norman M.
When did I begin?
Includes index.
1. Philosophical anthropology. 2. Embryology, Human. 3. Life–Origin.
I. Title.
BD450.F626 1988   129   88–7262

ISBN 0 521 34428 X hardback
ISBN 0 521 42428 3 paperback

CONTENTS

FOREWORD

It is a pleasure and a privilege to introduce Norman Ford's book. When I was chairman of the Committee of Enquiry on Human Fertilisation and Embryology, which reported in 1984, I tried hard to deter members of the Committee from asking the question When does Life Begin?. I thought it an ambiguous and misleading question. The answers to it could be unhelpfully various. Eggs, sperm, even individual cells, could all be said to be human and alive. As I saw it, we had to concentrate on the question when human life becomes morally and legally important. When do we have to ensure that human embryos are given the full protection of the law? At what stage in the development of the embryo should it be a criminal offence to use it for purposes of research? These were the pragmatic questions we tried to answer, in order to give advice to future legislators.

Norman Ford, in contrast, insists on raising the question when does an individual human being come into existence. He is interested in, and learned about, the old enigma of 'ensoulment'. But he is determined that the answers to such questions must be based on knowledge. He therefore examines the development of the human embryo immediately after fertilisation, using the knowledge that embryology now gives us.

As long as there is a possibility of two embryos, or none, developing from the loose conglomeration of cells that forms from the fertilised egg, he is not prepared to regard this conglomeration as a single entity. A singular noun is inappropriate for naming the collection of cells at this stage. He therefore cannot regard the pre-14-day embryo as a human individual. The answer to his question When did I begin? is '15 or so days from fertilisation'. It is at that stage that the human individual, of infinite worth, comes into existence.

I agree with his conclusion. But that is by the way. The true importance of Norman Ford's book lies in his determination to follow the argument wherever it leads: to search out and pursue the truth. His principle is that we must find out, as far as possible, where the truth lies, and then make moral sense of what we find. He succeeds in doing this. The spirit of courage, honesty and moral integrity shines through his book. It is a work of great significance, both for now and for the future.

Mary Warnock

PREFACE

1   Why did I write this book?

As a lecturer in moral philosophy and in the philosophy of the human person, it has always been important for me to know when a human person begins. In cases of rape it was necessary to know how long after the attack it was morally permissible to attempt to prevent a human embryo originating as a result of violence. This knowledge was crucial in differentiating morally between actions that prevented conception and those whose effect was really abortifacient. It became more pressing for me to be sure of my grounds on this issue once the freezing of human embryos began in some programmes of *in vitro* fertilization. Community debates in the media on the moral status of the human embryo convinced me of the necessity to inquire further into this question. Living in Melbourne provided the motivation and opportunities to learn the relevant scientific facts of early human embryology for a proper philosophical consideration of the question.

I had always believed, and taught for over 15 years, the commonly held traditional view that a human person begins once the process of fertilization is completed, i.e. once the pronuclei of the sperm and egg mix together. This gives rise to a single-cell human embryo, a zygote, whose genetic individuality and uniqueness remain unchanged during normal development. From that point on, cell divisions and differentiation are programmed for the organization and growth of the same developing human individual already present in the zygote. From the outset, the intrinsic unity of being in the embryo is evidenced by its unidirectional development and growth as one and the same living human being. According to this account the zygote is an actual human individual and not simply a potential human person in much the same way as an infant is an actual human person with potential to develop to maturity and not just a potential person. A person is an individual being. The zygote is an individual cell. It is easy to understand the zygote as a human individual with the potential to develop. Even when identical twinning happens, either the first human individual ceases when it divides and two new human individuals begin, or the original human individual continues when a newly formed twin begins. Identical twinning, of itself, does not in principle prove that the zygote could not be a human individual from the beginning. This view was in theory coherent but not necessarily correct; it was soon to be challenged on the grounds that it conflicted with newly discovered biological facts.

Though I had previously read arguments for delaying the beginning of human personhood for a couple of weeks, I was not convinced by the reasons adduced. My belief in the truth of the above account was first seriously shaken by the following extract from a letter by Professor Carl Wood published in the Melbourne newspaper *The Age* on 15 November 1982:

> The early embryo (up to eight cells) does have genetic individuality, but a multicellular individual is still not present. Two early embryos can be fused into one and one early embryo can divide into twins. Each cell behaves as if it is significantly independent of the other cells. Since persons, as usually defined, are multicellular individuals, it is difficult to maintain scientifically that a person has come into existence before the eight-cell stage. At least in a developmental sense, the early embryo is pre-individual.

It was this letter, with its hint of new evidence concerning the individuality of the early embryo that aroused my curiosity and triggered the absorbing research that eventually led me to write this book. For a few months I stopped researching because I was concerned my work would give the false impression that I favoured experimentation on human embryos. In this regard I stand by the latest teachings of the Catholic Church which shall be mentioned briefly towards the end of Chapter 2. I decided the right thing to do was to publish my findings as a responsible contribution to the search for the truth concerning when a human person begins. No long-term advantage is gained by suppressing the search for truth. In any case, a pro-life position cannot be effectively supported by dubious or false premises in relation to the beginning of the human person.

2 Methodology

The nature of this research was essentially inter-disciplinary, involving the disciplines of philosophy, scientific embryology and the history of both in relation to the beginning of the human individual. Tangentially, the history of the question did also touch on theological topics. Those interested in studying these topics would need to become acquainted with both philosophy and science. Few philosophers would be acquainted with early human embryology and few scientists would feel at home with philosophy. Many inter-disciplinary problems are touched on, but not pursued with full vigour where this is not required to establish the central thesis of the book. I did not think I should attempt to write an elementary book on human embryology for the benefit of my philosopher readers. Such books already abound. It seemed preferable to explain the necessary philosophical concepts and principles that ought to be employed and apply them to the facts of early human embryology. In this way philosophers, clerics and theologians who had some knowledge of early human embryology would be able to follow my line of argument. Equally, doctors, embryologists, medical students, nurses and students of the biological sciences would be able to follow the philosophical reasonings, as they have been explained for their benefit. Longer notes were necessary in the historical chapter to cater for the needs of those who wanted more detailed information on philosophy or theology than I assumed my average reader would require. In general, I have tried to provide for the needs of my readers with more enquiring minds in the notes by way of precise references and more detailed treatment of issues under discussion. Problems are raised early in the book, even in the Preface, to acquaint the reader with the issues but not to solve them immediately. In this way I have tried to prepare the reader to grasp the application of the philosophical concepts to the biological evidence given in the final chapters in the hope that the solution I propose may be found persuasive in the end.

3 Outline of treatment

I shall now provide a brief outline of the leading ideas and arguments of the book chapter-by-chapter to facilitate the reading of what might otherwise prove difficult.

In the first chapter additional reasons are given for the need of this book. Government reports touching on human embryos have been unable to resolve when the human individual or person begins. Linguistic usage of terms such as human life, human being, conception, embryo, etc., have to be analysed to understand their original pre-scientific meanings, as well as their contemporary employment in ordinary discourse. More importantly, from this chapter it is necessary to realize that modern science is quite relevant to the resolution of this problem even though it more properly pertains to philosophical reasoning to determine questions about the meaning and beginning of human personhood. All the same, philosophical induction cannot proceed without basing its reasoning on the findings of modern embryology.

Any philosophical theory that places the beginning of the human person at fertilization needs to be examined if it appears to conflict with the facts of modern biology. It is the role of philosophy to provide theories and conclusions that fit and explain the facts. There is no need to be afraid of the facts of experience or sound scientific data in the quest to uncover the objective philosophical truth about the beginning of the human person. Traditionally held philosophical theories and assumptions must be abandoned once their factual presuppositions fail to provide them with adequate support. All the available evidence is to be assessed objectively without allowing oneself to be swayed from the truth by personal preferences that fail to satisfy the relevant criteria of truth.

For about two thousand years the opinions of Aristotle, the great Greek philosopher and naturalist, on the beginning of the human being were commonly held. Chapter 2 explains the historical and cultural impact of his views up to our times. The model of his thinking was that of a potter who uses clay as material to make a vase. He argued that the male semen had a special power residing in it, *pneuma*, to transform the menstrual blood, first into a living being with a vegetative soul after seven days, and subsequently into one with a sensitive soul 40 days after contact with the male semen. At some unspecified time after this, rational ensoulment occurred. Aquinas adopted Aristotle's theory but specified that rational ensoulment took place through the creative act of God to transform the living creature into a human being once it had acquired a sensitive soul. The first *conception* took place over seven days, while the second conception or complete formation of the living individual with a complete human nature lasted 40 days. The blood was always potentially a human being, but not an actual human being until the formative action of the semen's *pneuma* or *air* was completed and complemented by the creation of a rational soul which thereafter performed the functions of the former vegetative and sensitive souls. The soul is also called a *form* because it shapes or forms matter from within into a specific kind of material being.

In short, the rational soul enables matter to become a human being, an animated body, an embodied soul, a human person.

Harvey's experiments with deer in 1633 proved Aristotle's theory of human reproduction wrong, without himself finding a satisfactory explanation of human conception. The use of primitive microscopes coupled with a lively imagination and a desire to establish rational ensoulment at the very beginning led to claims that a completely formed miniature human being (*homunculus*) could be seen in the sperm head. After modern scientists discovered the process of fertilization most people took for granted that the human being, complete with a rational soul, began once fertilization had taken place. The Catholic Church in particular, not finding any positive answers to this question in the Bible, over the centuries has always adopted the commonly accepted well-informed opinion of the day. Her main concern in this regard is ever to teach and promote the respect and protection morally due to human life from its outset, whether it is already personal or not. Today she presupposes that the zygote is already a human being with personal life, but does not expressly teach this doctrine. In so doing she accepts the commonly held view. The Church is well aware that some scholars around the world are discussing the beginning of the human person in relation to the biological beginning of human life, the establishment of the new individual's genetic individuality and the requirement of continuity of ontological identity.

After the introduction to philosophical reflection in the previous historical chapter, the reader is well prepared in Chapter 3 to confront the central philosophical concepts that need to be employed to determine what a human person is and when one begins. In the human person, soul and matter are one, constituting the characteristic psychosomatic unity of the human individual, a living human body and a unique ontological entity. It is not a question of finding out when a human individual begins to have personal experiences of his or her worth, or begins to be a moral agent after attaining the age of reason. It is not simply a matter of establishing when each one's genetic individuality begins. It is well known this occurs at fertilization. It is more a matter of finding out how far we can trace back our own personal identity as the same continuing individual living body, being or entity. This is what is meant by the ontological individuality or identity of a living person. An ontological individual is a distinct being that is not an aggregate of smaller things nor merely a part of a greater whole. Although the millions of cells in our bodies are genetically identical, each one is not an ontological individual or separate entity. There is only one human individual that really exists in the primary sense of actual existence, though there are many cells that share in the existence of that single living ontological individual. A human person is a distinct living ontological individual with a truly human nature. A human person cannot exist before the formation of a distinct living ontological individual with a truly human nature that retains the same ontological identity throughout successive stages of development. In this sense we judge that the adult is the same ontological individual as the child, the infant and even the fetus prior to birth. It will be necessary to consider the relevant embryological facts before determining that stage in embryological development before which there could not be an individual living body with a truly human nature that retains the same ontological identity from that point onwards.

Chapter 4 attempts to relate these philosophical concepts and principles to the biological data of human generation or reproduction. I have already presented the case for the commonly held view that the human individual begins when the zygote is formed at fertilization. Persuasive philosophical arguments, based on scientific evidence, suggest that this could not be so. We should not *a priori* and uncritically accept that because human genetic individuality is established from the zygote stage onwards, the zygote itself is a human individual. Human genetic individuality is not to be confused with human ontological individuality.

We need to see if the ontological individuality or identity of the zygote is retained from the first mitotic division onwards. The fact that identical twinning may occasionally occur at the zygote stage when it divides into the first two daughter cells raises a difficulty for the zygote being a human individual. If the zygote is a person, which of the two identical daughter cells is the original person when twinning occurs at that stage? Logic and common sense would favour saying two new human individuals begin in that case. The argument can be taken further. Every zygote has the capacity or potential to form twins at that stage. In other words, every human zygote, in the hypothesis under consideration, would be a human individual because of its central organization and capacity to continue as the same ontological individual until the adult stage. At the same time, and by the same token, each zygote could be regarded as two human individuals, because it also has the capacity to become two human individuals. How could a zygote be one distinct human individual whilst it still had the capacity to become more than one distinct individual? It might be said a cutting from a tree, once planted in the soil, may give rise to another tree without prejudice to the fact a tree was there in the first place. The short answer is that a tree is not a human zygote or a human individual. The biological structures of the tree and the human zygote reveal the essential differences that are relevant to determining whether one living individual continues in being or whether two new ones begin. The single-cell human zygote does not seem to be the same ontological individual as either one or both of its daughter cells. The evidence does not seem to support the required continuity of ontological identity from zygote to early embryo, and much less from zygote to fetus, infant, child and adult.

In Chapter 5 a similar case is argued, based on identical twinning occurring up to about 14 days after fertilization. It should not be assumed that a genetically unique human zygote is the same ontological individual as the resulting blastocyst, definitive embryo proper, fetus and child, notwithstanding the continuity of the same biological identity at every stage of development. Human twins that are genetically identical are nevertheless different ontological individuals. Furthermore, analysis of the evidence shows that early embryonic cells inside the zona pellucida lack the requisite unity to constitute a single ontological entity. Each is totipotent. They appear to have too much independence of behaviour to constitute one individual. This alone would preclude them from being a human individual until the multiplying cells formed themselves into a single multicellular human body. Furthermore, experiments with mice show how single cells taken from three separate early mouse embryos can be aggregated to form a single viable chimaeric mouse embryo. In this case the resultant individual mouse certainly did not begin at the zygote stage. This suggests that perhaps in the normal situation the proliferating and developing cells amalgamate at a later stage to form the definitive individual body, be it that of a mouse or a human individual.

All during the morula stage and prior to the early blastocyst stage the developing cells have not yet differentiated sufficiently to determine which cells will form the extraembryonic membranes (e.g. placenta) and those which will form the inner cell mass, from which will develop the embryo proper and fetus. Animal experiments show that by the late blastocyst stage when the inner cell mass is already formed, it is not yet determined which cells will give rise to the definitive embryo proper that will develop and grow into the fetus. It is argued a human individual cannot be present before it is actually formed. The traditional insight over the centuries remains ever valid: a potential human individual cannot be an actual human individual. There can be no person before the actual formation of a human individual, beginning as an on-going distinct individual embryonic human body.

Chapter 6 attempts to give an answer to when a human individual begins after stressing some differences between the development of eutherian mammals and amphibians. The former first need to form the placenta before forming the embryo proper, while the latter have no such need. With the appearance of the primitive streak after the completion of implantation and about 14 days after fertilization identical twinning can no longer occur. This is when the human body is first formed with a definite body plan and definitive axis of symmetry. Prior to this stage it would seem to be quite unreal to speak of the presence of a distinct human individual. This suggests that before this time genetically human embryonic cells could not develop into a human individual with a true human nature and a continuing ontological identity. If I am right, the early embryonic human cells could not constitute an actual human individual. Instead they would have the potency to form one or more human individuals. It seems that the biological evidence leads to the philosophical conclusion that a human individual, our youngest neighbour and member of the human community, begins at the primitive streak stage and not prior to it, but most certainly by the stage of gastrulation when the human embryo's primitive cardiovascular system is already functioning and blood is circulating.

4   Acknowledgements

It would not have been possible for me to attempt this project without the expert tuition, advice and constant encouragement from both Dr Alan Trounson, and Professor Roger Short in particular, who read and commented on several drafts of the text. I am most grateful to them for so generously giving me their time and sharing their knowledge with me whilst urging me at the same time to adhere to the teachings of my own Church. I am also indebted to Professor Carl Wood, Professor Robert MacMahon, Dr Shaun Brennecke, Dr Marie Dziadek and Dr Jeff Mann for their support and helpful criticisms of parts of my manuscript. I especially appreciated the valuble suggestions of Dr Anne McLaren and Professor John Hearn, who read the text in draft form. With the support of all the above experts in the biological sciences I felt I could confidently tackle the philosophical aspects of the conception and beginning of the human individual.

I am most grateful for the encouragement received over the last four years from the Rev. Dr Francis Moloney S.D.B., a member of the Vatican's International Theological Commission, and for his comments after reading the final draft of the text. I also thank the Rev. James

Acreman S.D.B., Rev. Max Grabau, the Rev. Dr John Begley S.J. and the Rev. Dr Thomas Daly S.J. for their helpful criticisms of my first draft. It goes without saying that I cannot claim they share all my views expressed in the final draft. I am most appreciative to Sr Therese Farrell, O.L.S.H., and Sr Margaret Bentley, F.M.A. for their help in improving the language, style and presentation of the text. In particular I am indebted to Dr Robin Pellew for his much appreciated support in the publishing of this book and to Ms Sheila Shepherd for her invaluable suggestions. I am most grateful to Mrs Susan Drew for her kindness, understanding and patience in typing all five drafts and the final copy of the text. Finally, I would like to thank the many publishers and authors for permission to reproduce some of their material, diagrams and photos.

My last and special word of thanks must be reserved to Baroness Warnock for kindly obliging to write a foreword for my book. Though our general philosophical outlooks differ in so many significant ways, we do share a common interest in the central themes of this book and substantially agree on the answer given to the question in its title – *When Did I Begin?*

Salesian Theological College
Oakleigh, Victoria, Australia
April 1987

1

Introduction

1 Interest in the beginning of the human individual: the purpose of this book

From time immemorial, people have been fascinated about the origin of the human race. Ancient myths abound. The *Genesis* story of Adam and Eve is known well enough. That is how the Bible represents the beginning of the human race through the direct creative intervention of God. If all we knew was that God created man and woman with the same human nature, we ourselves might not do much better than the author of *Genesis* when it came to depicting how this might have happened.

The theory of evolution presented a challenge to science as well as to the imagination when it was a question of explaining exactly how the first humans appeared on earth. A greater challenge was presented to philosophers and theologians when, without prejudice to their belief in the creation of the soul, they had to explain how, in pre-historic times, animal life could have been transformed into human life, a human being, a *Homo*. The term *hominization* was coined to refer to this process. The enormous leap beyond animal consciousness to typical human rational self-consciousness could only have occurred in virtue of the presence and functioning of a rational life-principle or soul. It is the soul that constitutes matter into a living human individual. Being animated by such a spiritual soul would have sufficed to change a form of animal life into a human being. Signs of this newly acquired, reflective self-awareness would have provided sufficient empirical evidence to convince any reasonable observer that the momentous change of *hominization* had occurred. A low degree of intelligence in the newly formed human being would have been irrelevant. Heated debates focused on how human individuals could derive from forms of animal life instead of being created instantly from the slime of the earth. It seemed the discussions only concerned remote events that must have occurred millions of years ago.

We are confronted with a similar problem if we consider precisely when each one of us began as an individual, whenever that moment may have been. One thing is certain – each one of us did come into existence by becoming a human being from something else. There was a point in time when we did not exist, except perhaps as a twinkle in our parents' eyes. Equally certain, there was another point in time when each of us did begin to be, though we cannot remember the moment, nor were we conscious at the time. Human beginnings, our beginnings, remain something of a mystery but they never cease to lose their fascinating appeal. We are ever curious about them. In particular, we would all like to know when we began to be human individuals. Most of us dismiss this as an impossible question to answer with any plausibility beyond an educated guess. I believe the time is ripe to search anew for an answer to this baffling question. It would need to be an answer that is obtained in the light of the scientific evidence available today as well as one that is able to withstand the critical probes of historical, linguistic and philosophical analysis. It is my hope that this book will suggest a reasonable solution to the riddle of when each of us began.

There are sufficient theoretical reasons to warrant pursuing an answer to this fascinating question for its own sake. It would be quite erroneous to confuse an interest in knowing when a human being begins with little regard for the proper respect and protection due to the early human embryo. The desire to know the plain truth would justify any energies spent in researching the beginning of the human individual. It is no trivial pursuit to investigate when the subject of a new personal existence actually begins, endowed by the Creator, as believers hold, with a destiny for eternal life and happiness.

Following recent developments in contraceptive techniques and especially in the treatment of infertility by *in vitro* fertilization, the question of when the human individual begins has also become an important practical issue. This practical interest derives from the bearing the answer to this question has on many moral problems. This is clear, for example, if one considers the relationship between when the human individual begins and the prevention of conception in the treatment of victims of rape within hours or days after the crime. In regard to the use of the intra-uterine device (I.U.D.) or the 'morning after pill' as contraceptives, it is important to know when a human individual begins if one wishes to avoid the risk of terminating the lives of embryonic human beings by performing acts with possible abortifacient effects. The same applies to the morality of some *in vitro* fertilization procedures, such as the deliberate discarding or freezing of human embryos and experimenting on them. These cases give rise to more significant moral objections if there is reason to believe that the early human embryo is already a human individual from the time of fertilization.

Heated public debates have taken place around the world on the morality of these and similar procedures, precisely because of the respect due to the human embryo from conception. There would be quite a difference in degree of moral malice between deliberately terminating the life of a human being at the embryonic stage and deliberately destroying cells that are not yet a human being but are destined to become one in a matter of hours or days. These are not idle theoretical matters. Legislators framing laws to regulate new reproductive technologies cannot avoid facing the crucial question of when human individuals begin. They have been caught unprepared for these developments. It is inevitable that the law will lag somewhat behind society's needs since it cannot readily proceed in advance of public opinion. The problems are difficult but they will not blow away. We cannot bury our heads in the sand. The pressing challenge of enquiring into our human beginnings needs to be taken up urgently. I hope to make a contribution to this discussion in this book and enable questions arising from a consideration of the moral status of human embryos to be answered with a due sense of responsibility.

The principal purpose of this book is to try to determine when a human individual begins. If this proves to be too difficult, we might have to settle for a specific stage in the reproductive process before which it would be impossible to say with any plausibility that a human individual exists. We certainly do begin to exist as human individuals at some stage. After all, a birthday is celebrated in the firm belief that the one who was born years ago is the same one who is presently celebrating the happy event. This same individual would be a human being, a member of the species *Homo sapiens*, a human person. While the thread of life is continuous from one generation to the next, human individuals certainly do begin and cease to exist in our world of experience.

Morality and the law dictate what ought to be done or omitted in relation to a human individual, but they do not determine what constitutes a human individual. This is presupposed. We can readily identify a child and a dog. Our attitudes towards them differ because we recognize that the child is a personal being that is superior to the dog in nature and dignity. Our attitudes and feelings do not make the child human. On the contrary, we respond to the recognition of the child's human nature and personal dignity by our attitudes of respect and love. Indeed, our conscience reproves us when we fail to respond to the presence of a human individual with the appropriate attitudes of respect, care and love. I believe it is possible and proper to treat separately the question of the origin of the human individual without necessarily dealing with the related important legal and moral implications of the answer given.

2   Moral status of the human embryo in government reports

Public concern about the fate of early human embryos during *in vitro* fertilization procedures has prompted several Government inquiries, in view of their special status. The United Kingdom committee was chaired by Baroness Mary Warnock, a distinguished philosopher, whose name now identifies both the committee and its report. The *Report of the Committee of Inquiry into Human Fertilisation and Embryology* was presented to Parliament in July 1984. There was no unanimity expressed on the degree of respect due to the early human embryo. The different views of the members of the Warnock Committee reflected those of the community. However, the Committee agreed it was unable to discriminate adequately between the moral status of the human individual or person and what constitutes a human individual and when this takes place during the continuous developmental process. The Warnock Report clearly states:

> Although the questions of when life or personhood begin appear to be questions of fact susceptible of straightforward answers, we hold that the answers to such questions in fact are complex amalgams of moral and factual judgements. Instead of trying to answer these questions directly, we have therefore gone straight to the question of *how it is right to treat the human embryo*. We have considered what status ought to be accorded to the human embryo, and the answer we give must necessarily be in terms of ethical or moral principles.[1]

Three members of the Committee in an expression of dissent showed how superficial their concept of person was by denying that the question of the beginning of a person was one of fact:

> 'When does the human person come into existence?' This cannot be answered in a simple fashion either. The beginning of a person is not a question of fact but of decision made in the light of moral principles. The question must therefore be refined still further. It

thus becomes 'At what stage of development should the status of a person be accorded to an embryo of the human species?' Different people answer this question in different ways. Some say at fertilisation, others at implantation, yet others at a still later stage of development. Scientific observation and philosophical and theological reflection can illuminate the question but they cannot answer it.[2]

The Warnock Report did not recognize the human embryo as a human being or a person. However, it did go so far as to state categorically:

> The status of the human embryo is a matter of fundamental principle which should be enshrined in legislation. *We recommend that the embryo of the human species should be afforded some protection in law.*[3]

In Australia the Victorian Government appointed Professor Louis Waller to chair *The Committee to Consider the Social, Ethical and Legal Issues Arising from In Vitro Fertilization.* Its final report was tabled in Parliament in August 1984 – *Report on the Disposition of Embryos Produced by In Vitro Fertilization.* It likewise failed to address itself to the questions of when an individual human being actually begins or the precise moral status of the early embryo. While it did not concede the human embryo is a human being or a person, the Waller Report did not regard the human embryo as an object or mere property:

> The Committee does not regard the couple whose embryo is stored as owning or having dominion over that embryo. It considers that these concepts should not be imported into and have no place in a consideration of issues which focus on an individual and genetically unique human entity.[4]

The reference to 'human entity' does not indicate that the Waller Committee regards the product of fertilization as a human being. The choice of language is deliberately vague without any attempt being made to be philosophically precise.

The Waller Committee recommended that research on embryos be limited to excess embryos. The reasons given for this majority decision are as follows:

> These members consider that formation of embryos solely for research or experimentation is not acceptable in Victoria today. From a moral perspective, it may be said that, regardless of the particular level of respect which different sections of the com-

munity would accord an embryo, this individual and genetically unique human entity may not be formed *solely* and from the outset to be used as a means for any other human purpose, however laudable.[5]

In 1985 Senator Brian Harradine introduced a private member's Bill in the Australian Senate to prohibit destructive non-therapeutic experimentation on human embryos. After it had passed its second reading, the Senate appointed a seven-member Senate Select Committee to consider various aspects of the Harradine Bill in relation to experimentation on human embryos in the context of *in vitro* fertilization. Under the chairmanship of Senator Tate, the Committee was named the *Senate Select Committee on the Human Embryo Experimentation Bill 1985*. Its Report was presented to the Australian Senate on 8 October 1986 after having studied 270 submissions from all over Australia and heard evidence from a total of 64 witnesses. The Report and the nine published volumes of evidence heard by the Senate Committee demonstrate how seriously the Senate members took their task. Central to their deliberations and recommendations was the moral status of the early human embryo and the determination of when a human being begins.

The Senate Committee was well aware of the various international medical conventions that outline ethical guidelines for experimentation on human subjects, human beings or persons. In its own words:

> ...the Committee has not attempted to attribute the status of 'person' to the embryo in either its philosophical or legal senses. It does not intend to pronounce on this question....[6]

At the same time the Senate Committee believed that the ethical principles that apply to experimenting on human subjects are also relevant in the case of experimenting on human embryos for the simple reason that:

> ...the Committee was not persuaded that similar principles regulating destructive non-therapeutic experimentation should not apply to the embryo regarded as genetically new human life organised as a distinct entity oriented towards further development. No marker event advanced carried such weight that different principles should apply to distinguish the fertilised ovum from that which all would agree is a human subject.[7]

The Senate Committee considered various stages in the development of the embryo from fertilization onwards, but was unable to be satisfied that any particular one was decisive for establishing a point prior to which the developing embryo could not be regarded as a human being. The Committee succinctly summed up its position as follows:

> In this situation prudence dictates that, until the contrary is demonstrated 'beyond reasonable doubt' (to use an expression well known in our community), the embryo of the human species should be regarded as if it were a human subject for the purposes of biomedical ethics.[8]

The Committee immediately added another paragraph in which it admitted the possibility that this situation could change in the future:

> The Committee is not precluding the possibility of such a marker event being so made out with the degree of certainty indicated, but it advises the Senate that no such compelling evidence is forthcoming at the time of preparing this Report.[9]

In the final analysis, the Senate Select Committee, even though unable to resolve the question of the personal status of the human embryo, preferred:

> ...to regard the embryo not as 'property belonging to', but as an entity enjoying the protection of a guardian. Under this model the property rights of gamete donors are exhausted on fertilisation when a genetically unique new human life organised as a distinct entity oriented towards further development comes into being. At that point guardianship arises....[10]

Government Committees of Inquiry into the social, legal and ethical issues arising from new human reproductive technologies are not necessarily the best qualified groups of persons to enquire into, and resolve, the philosophical question of the beginning of the human individual. This is why they failed to address the issue. It is more a theoretical philosophical problem than an ethical or legal one. Admittedly, scientific facts of embryology need to be presupposed. In the last analysis, however, the question is philosophical and can only be resolved fully by people with some acquaintance with philosophical concepts, reasoning and methods as well as the basic relevant facts of human embryology.

3   Problems of language

Peoples the world over have been speaking about conception and birth since the origin of human language. The word *conceive* in the various languages acquired its meaning hundreds and perhaps thousands of years ago when very little human reproductive biology was known and when the processes of reproduction were shrouded in myth and mystery. The choice of the term was made on the basis of the knowledge available to indicate simply that a woman was pregnant and was soon to become a mother by giving birth to a child growing in her womb. This much could be known without any scientific knowledge of human reproduction. The term *'conceive'* acquired its original popular meaning in this way without any suggestion as to how or when a new life began, apart from being the consequence of sexual intercourse. Observational and common-sense criteria guided human perception in this sphere in various places and cultures. The language employed was sufficiently clear and precise to satisfy the ordinary requirements of communication to signify that a woman had succeeded in becoming pregnant and that a fetus or child had begun to exist and grow. This is the essence of what was meant by the ideas and the terms used to express the popular perceptions of conception and pregnancy.

The original meaning of the English word *conceive* refers to a woman receiving the seed in her womb and becoming pregnant by taking the fetus to herself. This is the essence of the active meaning of conception. The English word has the primary meaning of 'to take effectively, take to oneself, take in and hold'.[11] The word *conceive* comes from the Latin *concipere* whose general meaning is 'to take or lay hold of, to take to oneself, to take in, take, receive, etc.'[12] Its biological meaning is 'to take or receive (animal or vegetable) fecundation, to conceive, become pregnant'.[13] The simple primitive insight expressed by *conception* is that of a female mammal holding on to the semen which in some mysterious way leads to the start of a new life and thereby enables her to bear offspring in her womb. The passive meaning of conception refers to the child or offspring being created or formed in the womb and thereby beginning to exist. In this latter sense the emphasis is on the origin of the child rather than the action of the mother.

The Greek term κυέω (kueō) means 'to bear in the womb, to be pregnant with, to be formed, to be big, to conceive'.[14] κύημα (kuēma) is derived from this term and means 'that which is conceived, embryo, fetus'.[15] Another Greek word used is συλλαμβάνω (sullambanō). Its basic meaning is similar to the Latin, namely, 'collect, gather together, lay hands on, seize, receive at the same time and, of females, conceive'.[16] The ordinary Hebrew word for conceive or become pregnant is 'hārāh'.[17] There is another word 'yāham' that is usually used in reference to cattle coming into oestrus and means 'to be hot, to conceive'. No doubt this term refers to the sexual impulse of animals at the time of breeding – heat being taken as the cause of conception.[18]

The Chinese use a Cantonese expression pronounced 'why young' which means 'to nurture in the womb' to convey the notion of conception. It is interesting to note that the character for 'womb' is a composite one denoting a 'child that is starting or growing'.[19] The Japanese expression 'haramu' is a traditional one that refers to the state or condition of being pregnant and means 'to be swollen with child'.[20] There is another more technical Japanese expression 'jutai' whose meaning is 'to receive a child in the womb'.[21] The ancient Vietnamese term for conception is 'có mang' which means 'to be pregnant', where 'mang' means 'fetus in the womb'.[22] There is another common Vietnamese expression 'mang thai'; 'to conceive, to be pregnant with child',[23] where 'mang' means 'carry or bear' and 'thai' means 'fetus in the womb'. A more literary expression is 'thu thai' which means 'to conceive, to become pregnant', 'to receive and flourish with a baby in the womb.'[24] It is interesting to note that in China, Japan and Vietnam, a child was traditionally considered to be one year old on the day of birth. Consideration of the Chinese year apart, one reason for this custom could possibly be to give recognition to the time spent in one's mother's womb from conception to birth.

The word *embryo* in English is a corruption of the Latin *embryon*, itself an ancient English word also believed to be derived from the Greek ἐν 'in' + βρύειν 'to swell, to grow'.[25] In this sense embryo would have meant 'the one swelling or growing inside'. The Greek word ἔμβρυον primarily means 'the young one' and its second meaning is embryo or fetus.[26] The original sense of ἔμβρυον is to be found in its root term βρύω meaning 'swell or teem with', 'to be full of', 'abound, grow luxuriantly', 'burst forth with'.[27] The original perception amongst the Greeks referred to 'the young one swelling or growing in the womb'. It is helpful to bear in mind this original derivation of the term *embryo* from the pre-cellular theory times when it is presently applied to the first cells from which the mature mammal develops. For the Greeks the embryo results from conception and refers to what is conceived and is beginning to swell or grow as a young one in the womb. They entirely lacked the modern notion of 'fertilization'.

This brief survey shows that when the various linguistic expressions for conception in the active sense were formed, there was no concern for indicating exactly how or when a human individual came into existence after the act of sexual intercourse, other than to signify that the woman had begun to be pregnant. A pregnancy that is recognized after the first missed menses, which is the usual clinical sign that a woman may be pregnant, is called a 'clinical pregnancy'. Subsequently this may be confirmed by a medical examination. Traditionally this would have been the first hint to a woman that she may be pregnant. By this time implantation would have normally been completed, two weeks after fertilization. Nowadays a pregnancy may be recognized after implantation has begun but before the first missed menses. This is known as a 'biochemical pregnancy' since it can only be diagnosed by the presence of a hormone called chorionic gonadotrophin (CG) found in the blood or urine some 6–9 days after fertilization. This human chorionic gonadotrophin (hCG) is secreted by the tropoblastic cells of the conceptus as implantation is beginning. A positive result of the test may be mistaken if the trophoblast develops without an inner cell mass or subsequent embryo and fetus.

When conception is used passively, it refers to the beginning of the human being's existence without indicating the precise moment when that occurs in terms of any biological process or event. It is not hard to see how in common estimation the timing of the occurrence of conception in the active and passive meanings could easily be identified. In this way one could say: 'When my mother conceived *me* she was in Melbourne.' Yet if pressed by objections, one would hardly concede that the mere linguistic use of this proposition would commit one philosophically to the identification in time of the two senses of conception. Nevertheless, we must admit that cultural attitudes and common traditional beliefs have been powerfully influenced by our ordinary pre-scientific perceptions and linguistic usage in regard to human conception.

Over the last hundred years or so, the process of fertilization has become to be identified with conception in the view of most people. Hence fertilization, almost universally, has acquired the cultural heritage and status of conception itself, particularly in its passive sense. The problem remains because many do not believe this should be so, especially among scientists and philosophers. They wish to challenge the legitimacy of such an easy and almost semantic inheritance of the status of a human individual by mere ordinary linguistic usage.

Linguistic forms depend on common usage, which in turn depends on our ordinary needs for communicating information to one another. Until recently there was little need to distinguish in practical life between the beginning of fertilization and the end of the process. Ordinary language has no word to refer to such intermediate states of being. Now it is crucial to give a legal definition of the meaning of 'embryo' with reference to the process of fertilization in the context of clarifying the limits of legally permitted research on human embryos. While this shows the limitations of ordinary language for scientific purposes, it also highlights the culturally determining influence of terms such as *embryo* coined in the age of pre-scientific knowledge of human reproductive biology.

When a human ovum is fertilized by a human sperm a new individual living cell originates that can be said to have human life. It is called human life because it results from the fusion of human gametes. It is also called human life because an adult human being can certainly be derived from it. The question is whether the fertilized egg or progenitor human cell is already a human being. There are two human lives since both mother and the embryo are alive. Its life is certainly distinct from the life of the mother, though it is initially very much dependent on her for continuing existence and support. IVF embryos are alive but die unless they are implanted in the mother's womb. This human life could very well be an individual human being, a person – but this cannot be taken for granted.

There is a further problem of language to be resolved in relation to the expression 'human life'. In many contexts it quite unambiguously refers to a human individual or human being. This need not necessarily be so. In the case of the transplantation of a live human heart or kidney, we are dealing with live human organs: they have *human* life but they are not human individuals or human beings. They are certainly not canine or feline forms of life. They are referred to as having human life because they come from human beings. Thus we certainly cannot equate the expression 'human life' with 'human being'. The same could be said about a live human ovum and a live human sperm. They are a form of human life but they are not human beings.

There is one final problem of language that can cause conceptual confusion. People often use the expressions 'human individual' and 'human being' as inter-changeable or equivalent. I think this can be fairly assumed in ordinary discourse but not necessarily so on the lips of all philosophers. In ordinary usage every human individual and every human being is understood to be a human person. While I believe this is true, I admit further philosophical clarification and arguments are needed, as we shall see in Chapter 3. Human personhood is definitely a philosophical concept and as such eludes adequate investigation by empirical sciences. Though it is agreed that all human persons are human individuals there is no unanimity that all human individuals are also human persons.

Our use of language needs to be analysed in order to clarify these concepts as well as their relationships among themselves. This should be done if we are to arrive at a satisfactory answer to the question of when a human individual begins. There is no need to inquire exhaustively into the philosophy of the human person and all its ramifications. We simply need to establish the necessary and sufficient criteria for determining when a human person or human individual begins.

4   Considerations of method

(i)   *A case for philosophical induction*

Many philosophical questions are resolved following the analytical method of reasoning, deducing conclusions from general premises. We can conclude that God does not have dimensions once it is known that He is non-material since non-material beings are not bodies that can be measured. Once we know that an animal is a mother, we can deduce that it is a female. Again it can be known by deduction that one who is certainly a moral agent, must be already capable of exercising self-conscious and free acts.

Not all truths, however, can be found out in this way. The employment of the inductive method of reasoning, with keen attention given to experience and observation, is required to establish some facts or some general truths that depend on factual situations. Induction often involves inferences from facts to general principles. Many philosophical truths can only be established inductively after a careful assessment of all the available relevant evidence. It is only after thinking inductively in the light of well-founded philosophical principles that we can come to discover whether some of our sense-perceptions are misleading, whether the world of our experience consists of one or many really distinct things or beings, whether God exists, whether evolution is possible and/or probable, whether we can personally survive after death and whether particular acts are immoral. It is also only through the philosophical use of inductive reasoning that we can successfully arrive at sound conclusions concerning the beginning of human individuals.

Deductive reasoning is either valid or invalid. Inductive thinking admits of various degrees of support for a conclusion according to whether it is based on evidence that is weak, good or conclusive. Think for a moment of how carefully a detective weighs all the evidence when trying to solve a crime. The number of suspects is gradually narrowed down when the evidence supporting a particular solution mounts and becomes fairly conclusive. A jury uses the same type of inductive reasoning when it deliberates a verdict during a trial. It convicts only when it is convinced beyond reasonable doubt that the accused is guilty according to the law, solely on the basis of the evidence presented to it. Rulings can be given regarding the admissibility of certain evidence, but not regarding the evaluation of the evidence made during the jury's deliberations. The weighing and assessing of the worth of evidence is the responsibility of the jury. The verdict simply expresses the conclusion of a process of induction – assertion or denial that the evidence was found convincing beyond reasonable doubt.

In a similar way the conclusions of all inductive reasonings are reached on the grounds of the evidence interpreted in the light of one's common sense, general experience of life, cultural outlook and conceptual framework. The same dynamics are at work in cases of inductive thinking in the philosophical sphere. Of paramount importance for the outcome of philosophical inductive reasoning is one's more or less implicit metaphysical presuppositions. It makes a world of difference whether one's basic philosophical position does, or does not, allow for objects that do not lie within the bounds of our possible experience. While it is true that all would agree that we can explain a human individual's life in terms of observable processes, phenomena and functions, not all would agree that such an explanation would be complete without allowing for some non-empirical, non-observable, but nonetheless real principle of life or soul that would account for its unity in being, directive organic activities and reflective self-conscious acts. There is to be no arbitrary restricting of the conceptual framework within which philosophical inductive thinking is to be carried out.

This point is worth pursuing because it does influence the philosophical conclusions drawn from an analysis of biological facts learnt through experience. All our concepts ultimately originate from our experience in the sense that they cannot be meaningful unless they relate in some way to concepts formed by the application of empirical criteria. Human experience, coupled with the use of empirical criteria, must be the absolute referring point for the source of meaningfulness for all human thinking and its expressions in language. But this does not imply that all the concepts employed in our thinking are limited to objects of possible experience.

Our concepts are derived from empirically observable situations, find their original home there and are unambiguously employed in the world of everyday experience. This does not provide any justification for labelling their employment as meaningless when empirical criteria are not, or could not be, available for their application. To claim that all non-empirical employment of our concepts distorts them is to disregard how we do successfully employ some concepts in non-empirical ways in meaningful discourse. It would be over playing one's hand to rule out non-empirical concepts as meaningless when one has gratuitously adopted an empirical principle of significance for the meaningful use of all concepts.[28] Likewise, there can be no justification for unreasonably limiting the meaning or validity of 'proof' to instances where only empirical criteria of significance are employed. No doubt those who do admit the meaningful use of non-empirical concepts may often disagree among themselves over the claims of any particular philosophical conclusion to have sufficient inductive support to warrant drawing any conclusions with certainty.

We have seen how different philosophical presuppositions could significantly influence our interpretation of biological facts. This is particularly so when we are considering the beginning of the human individual or the human person. But not only theoretical or philosophical views can affect the outcome of the conclusion of inductive thinking. One's final judgment may be unduly swayed, even subconsciously, by a variety of subtle factors of a non-theoretical or rather practical nature that are related to when a human individual begins (e.g. selfishness). Among such factors the following may be found on occasion: an uncritical acceptance of traditional beliefs and cultural assumptions, plain ignorance of biological facts, blind prejudice, a variety of emotional reactions to any suggestions of a need to revise one's personal views, a fear of undermining the moral stand against abortion and experimentation on human embryos, a utilitarian pro-abortion and pro-experimentation attitude in relation to human embryos and, finally, an unwillingness to come to grips with the social, political, legal and moral consequences of the emergence of the truth in relation to when human beings begin. Morality and social cohesion are promoted more by seeking and living out the truth than hiding and insulating oneself from it. We should do our best to be objective in searching for the truth even if there is no guarantee that we will fully succeed when we have to interpret and evaluate the facts. In any case, a responsible attempt at the philosophical determination of the beginning of the human individual should go ahead irrespective of the likely effects the answer given might have on some in the community.

(ii)   *Philosophical conclusions to be based on scientific embryology*

To avoid the danger of deducing *a priori* answers to our question from abstract metaphysical principles, we need to reflect seriously on the findings of the relevant empirical scientific disciplines, namely, human reproductive biology and embryology. Sound philosophical thinking can never proceed independently of ordinary human experience. Metaphysical theories must be based on facts, and in our case, embryological facts. All the required scientific evidence, including whatever can be drawn from experiments done with non-human embryos, should be given careful consideration. It is inconceivable that we should philosophically research into the origins of the human individual and by-pass the early relevant mammalian and human developmental stages from fertilization onwards.

It is quite arbitrary to think of the human individual only in terms of a later stage of development, namely, when self-consciousness has been acquired. Naturally, we begin our thinking about the origin of the human individual when we ourselves are quite mature, but we should not stop there. The evidence of early human development needs to be viewed in the light of general metaphysical principles and of the criteria required for the constitution of a human being, to determine, as best we can, the beginning of a human individual.

The empirical methods of science may provide the facts, but this does not imply that science alone can supply their ultimate significance in terms of the beginning of human individuality or human personhood. Biologists distinguish various stages of continuous development all through the human life span for practical and medical reasons, not to indicate the presence or absence of a human individual. One should not expect an embryologist to be able to say when a human individual begins to exist as distinct from indicating various stages of development in human repro-duction. Just as there can be no exclusive claim to human individuality or personhood on the grounds of race, sex, colour, intelligence, creed, or state of mental or physical health neither can there be by reason of any particular stage of development. Irrespective of age one either is or is not a human individual. The individual's life process is continuous from when the individual begins to exist. However, the human individual cannot be reduced to the status of a process. The living human individual is the subject of the life process, but not simply a process itself.

(iii)   *An inter-disciplinary task and its challenges*

The *inter-disciplinary* nature of the beginning of the human individual raises difficulties of its own as people are not usually well versed in the methodologies of both science and philosophy. Misunderstandings frequently occur in relation to terminology, facts and their interpretations. Doctors and scientists are quite competent to determine that the death of a person has occurred, especially brain death. Insuperable philosophical problems do not arise here. The cessation of the human life process marks the beginning of the presence of a corpse. Tissue death and the death of organs may take some time after brain death has occurred.[29] Nevertheless, at times errors have been made in declaring that death has taken place. Caution is needed in cases where doubts may arise.

Scientists do get entangled in philosophical snares when determining the beginning of human life. Life is a necessary condition for the presence of a human individual. This does not imply that doctors or scientists are competent to determine the moment of the beginning of the human individual. Scientifically determined irreversible absence of brain activity is a good indicator that death has already taken place at the end of the life continuum. Absence of brain electric activity in the early human fetus does not necessarily have the same significance because the embryo has the potential to develop right through to adulthood.[30] One cannot conclude from the absence of a human individual after brain death has occurred to the non-presence of a human individual or person prior to the first appearance of brain electric activity in the fetus. How the philosophical concept of potentiality is employed is of crucial significance in determining the beginning of the human individual. In this case it is the proper task of philosophers to explore the meaning and application of the notion of potentiality, together with its correlative notion of actuality. It will be difficult to draw the fine line between where the strictly scientific evidence ends and philosophical interpretation starts when it comes to determining when a human individual begins to exist.

Similar problems arise concerning the *soul* or human life-principle. Once death takes place we are quite certain the soul is no longer present in the corpse precisely because there are no longer signs of a life-principle in operation. Scientists are unable to observe the human soul since it is not a concrete object but a non-empirical life-principle and consequently is not directly detectable by scientific methods of observation. We can infer the spiritual soul is present when a child acquires the ability to predicate, to realize the meaning of truth and falsehood and to be capable of moral acts. In doing so we can hardly say we are relying entirely on direct empirical methods of research and understanding. Another difficult question to answer is whether one can be sure the spiritual soul is present before the obvious expressions of its presence are manifested through the incipient rational acts of the child at the onset of the age of reason. It is quite an important issue because many people believe a human individual could not be a human person unless he/she was animated by a spiritual or rational soul.

A further question that science alone cannot solve is whether there is any need to postulate a spiritual soul in the first place. Theists generally are agreed that the human person is animated by a spiritual soul, while non-believers and empiricists in general do not think there is sufficient evidence to support such a belief at all. These are all important inter-disciplinary issues that need to be dealt with in the course of establishing when a human individual or human person begins to exist.

Science and philosophy are both required for the *interpretation of the significance of natural purposes and directive activities* found in nature. At times these are clearly indicative of a variety of functions of a single organism. It is clear that various organs (e.g. heart, lungs, liver, senses etc) belong to one mammal and are designed to function for the benefit of the same mammal. The natural purpose of their functioning is to enable the organism to live. There are other acknowledged natural instances of directive and purposive activities in our world without the slightest suggestion that the world is a single organic individual entity. The relationships of the movements of the heavenly bodies in our solar system together with those of the seasons, the tides, days followed by nights and even of wet and dry weather indicate inter-dependence of natural systems rather than a one living organic universe. In other cases similar relationships are obvious signs of the existence of many inter-related organic individuals. Think of the significance and purpose of human sexuality, the mating habits of animals, the dependence of the young on their parents and social relations and collaboration in a hive of bees. Natural purposive inter-actions between living individuals serve the needs of many species.

Natural directive purposive activities are also found in the human reproductive process. It will be a very delicate inter-disciplinary problem to determine when these activities are signs of the presence of a new multicellular human individual and when they indicate purposive inter-actions between many living organisms and/or cells in a reproductive process that results in the formation of a new human individual. We need to be able to discriminate between the development of a multicellular human individual and a mass of genetically human cells in a process of developing into a multicellular human individual.

It would not be wise to attempt to answer the question: 'When does a human individual begin?' without considering the contributions made by previous generations. We stand to learn much from *history*. Our cultural perceptions of the beginning of the human individual have been moulded over the last two thousand years, especially during the last two centuries. It would be helpful to make a brief historical survey of the significant views that have dominated human perceptions over the centuries, explaining why these views were held and, more importantly, why they were changed. This will be an excellent introduction to the philosophical aspects of the problem while learning what is offered by the wisdom of the ages. It will prepare readers for a discussion of some of the contemporary issues as well as an understanding of the philosophical thinking underlying the line of argument adopted in this book. This in its turn will better equip us to examine the embryological evidence in the light of the relevant metaphysical principles and concepts that best seem both to respond to the facts and yet remain in harmony with a sound sense of realism.

An inter-disciplinary approach demands that positions be argued thoroughly without exaggerating their value. Inconclusive arguments need to be exposed, even if they happen to support one's conclusions. A case in point would be the argument that pre-implanted embryos could not be human individuals because their high wastage rate would conflict with the wisdom and goodness of a Provident Divine Creator. It is not at all helpful to rely on arguments that have some appeal but fail to convince or prove their point. Finally, it will be necessary to differentiate between evidence that is capable of giving strong or only weak support for conclusions reached in relation to when a human individual begins.

2

Historical influence of Aristotle on the theory of human reproduction

1   Why a return to Aristotle?

Aristotle was not only the greatest Greek biologist and philosopher, but also the most influential in our Western civilization. For about two thousand years, since his death in 322 B.C., his teachings have formed our traditional understanding of the origin of the individual human being. From the middle of the seventeenth century his views had been on the decline. Recently, however, there has been a revival of his theory in favour of delaying the origin of the individual human being for some weeks after conception.

This is a welcome revival for a variety of reasons. Aristotle knew how to harmonize his vast empirical observations, acquired as a naturalist and biologist, with the requirements of a philosophical interpretation of the same. There is no opposition between the facts as they were known in his day and his metaphysical categories and principles. His philosophy represents one of the best examples of common-sense realism. He did not merely observe developing parts and organs in a living creature – he interpreted them philosophically as parts and organs of one developing living being. Children know that an arm is not a leg. They also know that both an arm and a leg are equally parts of the one developing individual being. The viewpoints of biology, philosophy and ordinary experience are quite compatible – they should be seen as mutually complementing each other. Not every kind of philosophy is capable of succeeding here. The Aristotelian philosophical conceptual framework facilitates the formation of an integrated perspective.

Scientists have learnt from history to appreciate the evolutionary model of thinking for their own disciplines, society and the world at large. This helps us to understand our present position in so many spheres of intellectual endeavour. When it is a matter of grasping the origin of the human individual we cannot ignore the history of this subject. Our ideas and language about the beginning of the human individual have been moulded within the conceptual framework of Aristotle's biology and philosophy throughout Western civilization.

The historical evidence shows how opinions concerning when the human individual began changed over the centuries in accordance with how facts, or 'presumed facts', were interpreted through the prism of Aristotle's conceptual scheme. Much the same can be said of similar disagreements today. The correct way to go about resolving this ancient question is to approach the task as an inter-disciplinary one by combining the resources of history, philosophy and science.

Some scientists have recently been genuinely surprised by community concern about certain aspects of new reproductive technologies. This became obvious after the publishing of various government reports on the ethical, social and legal issues involved in *in vitro* fertilization and experimentation on human embryos. These reports merely voiced the ethical difficulties that arose from implicitly held philosophical beliefs and assumptions about when human beings begin. Whereas many in the community consider human embryos to be developing human beings, many scientists believe they are only clusters of dividing cells that could develop into human beings.

It is very easy for doctors and scientists to view organs and developing cells from an objective viewpoint that is purely empirical, as though this was the only way of viewing them. They need to bear in mind that the empirical approach is not the only way to find out objective truths about things in our world. Scientists and doctors should acknowledge that many ordinary people who are not scientists may objectively see things from both an empirical and a non-empirical perspective. This may be so even if they are unable to articulate their insights without some introduction to elementary philosophical concepts and principles of reasoning.

While the community should try to learn and appreciate what the scientists are saying and doing, scientists should try to understand why many in the community are alarmed about certain aspects of their work in the area of reproductive technology. This is all the more necessary if scientists are to enter into fruitful dialogue with the members of the broader community. Aristotle's approach to resolving the question of when a human being begins could provide some useful objective considerations that are not dependent on a particular religious belief. An acquaintance with his theory of human reproduction or generation would appear to be imperative for anybody who wishes to understand fully the crucial issues in the contemporary debates. While modern science has corrected Aristotle's biological errors, his philosophical principles remain valid when applied to the relevant facts of modern embryology.

Aristotle had a healthy respect for the things in this material world: they were not merely weak imitations of ideas that existed in the heavens as Plato believed. They were themselves genuine things, realities, both living and non-living beings. Knowledge of them could be obtained by observation. What Aristotle observed, however, was interpreted in accordance with the generally accepted philosophical principles of his time, especially those related to causation. While some philosophical presuppositions enable us to acquire a more comprehensive understanding of what is observed, other philosophical positions might inhibit our perception of certain empirical aspects to the detriment of a true knowledge of all the facts at hand. The reverse could also occur: false or inadequate biologial knowledge could lead one to adopt faulty philosophical premises.

In the light of this, it would be wise to start with a brief outline of some of Aristotle's general philosophical ideas on causes and change, the better to understand his biological and metaphysical account of the origin of the individual human being. He certainly learnt some embryological notions from his predecessors in the previous century, e.g. Empedocles (d. 444 B.C.) and Hippocrates (d. about 370 B.C.). To the extent that their views coincided with his, they are all included under the general heading of Aristotle's Theory of Human Generation or Reproduction.[1]

2   Philosophical underpinnings of Aristotle's theory of human reproduction

Aristotle's philosophy is often called metaphysics because he was most concerned with explaining the ultimate reasons or causes of the existence of concrete objects, i.e. individual material beings. Such an enquiry starts from empirical observations of bodies, but inevitably leads to considerations that are quite non-empirical in character in an attempt to plumb the depths of the meaning and causes of material beings and how it is possible for them to change from one type of material being to another. The original meaning of existence given in our experience is exemplified in bodies or particular material beings. They appear to be real *par excellence*: whatever else is real is considered so by reason of its positive relationship with individual bodies that primarily exist for us in the first instance. This immediately highlights levels of existence or reality within a single particular body. While a piece of wood is really existing in a concrete way, together with oxygen in the air, it is also able to become gases and ashes through combustion. Hence it is said to be *actually* a piece of wood, while at the same time it is *potentially* ashes and gases which may subsequently come into *actual* existence through combustion.

These two principles of *actuality* and *potentiality* are very important for understanding Aristotle's metaphysical philosophy. The wood *is* *actually* wood, not ashes and gases; but it *is potentially* ashes and gases. Through a process of change it can become something completely different. This example illustrates how these two principles work in relation to several separate individual bodies. They may also be applied to one and the same individual body that retains its own identity and existence while undergoing a change that merely modifies it. Water that is actually 20 degrees Celsius is also potentially 50 degrees Celsius. In the primary sense of the term *exists* it is still the *same water* notwithstanding a real change in temperature. It is obvious that potentiality and actuality are two really distinct principles of being that are required to explain levels of existence and change in individual bodies. They are not to be conceived as two separate beings or individual bodies within any one individual thing. They are two real principles of being that constitute a single body. However, it does belong to the identity of wood to have this potential or capacity to burn and thereby become ashes and gases. All this shows the fundamentally dynamic mutability of bodies or material beings in relation to existence at its various levels. A body is essentially mutable, because it has the potential to change and even become a different kind of body.

More is required if we are to explain the existence of particular material beings. Aristotle suggests *four causes*, each of which in a specific way influences the coming into being of a particular thing.[2] The first is called the *efficient* cause. This is the agent, e.g. the builder of a house, a sculptor or a potter. The efficient cause needs some direct or indirect contact with one or more bodies to set a process in motion that results in the production of something, frequently termed its effect. Though more easily grasped as a personal agent, the efficient cause may also be non-personal, e.g. the *sun* heating the earth, the *wind* felling a tree or a *dog* biting a child. The agent is active in relation to what it affects, causing it to passively undergo a change, whereby what was previously existing in potency is now actualized. A sculptor can change a marble block into a statue. The action of the efficient cause (sculptor) changes the marble from a potential statue into an actual statue. The efficient cause is always an actual being quite distinct from what it acts upon. It is outside or extrinsic to the being of the body or bodies produced or modified as a result of its action. The sculptor is not the marble or the statue.

A personal efficient agent has a reason, motive or purpose for acting. This is the *end* or *that on account of which* the efficient cause initiates a process of change. The builder's purpose is to produce a home to live in, just as an author hopes his writings will be published in a book. It is this purpose that motivates the agent, explaining *why* a particular process of activity starts in the first place. No rational agent acts without a purpose as our common experience and court proceedings at trials confirm. The purpose is referred to as the *final* cause. Again, in the case of personal agents it is clear the final cause is also extrinsic to the effect produced since the purpose is in the mind of the agent.

Aristotle also believed final causes are at work in natural processes, in-built into the dynamic infra-structure of all changes in nature. It is as though some plan, some rational design or purpose is being followed in natural processes, upon the achievement of which the process terminates. The natural processes involved in the gestation of a mammal stop once the offspring is born. This is so because the purpose of the processes of gestation is to give birth to live offspring, if all goes well. In this sense, purpose or the final cause enters into the meaning of a natural process.

Coming to the object produced we have two causes, namely, the *material* cause and the *formal* cause. These are *intrinsic*, i.e. accounting for the constitution of the very being of the object from within itself. Traditionally this has been known as the *hylomorphic* theory, from the Greek derivation literally meaning *matter–form* theory. The material cause is the underlying substratum from which an object is produced in a process initiated by the efficient cause. The house is made from wood, the statue from marble and the jar from clay. These materials *of themselves* are open to being fashioned into any shape or form by the agent in accordance with a given plan. This is why the material cause is said to be indeterminate in itself, receiving determination during the production process. The artist skilfully passes on the *form* or plan in mind to the marble when a statue is made. This is said to be the *formal* cause, the one that ultimately determines the actual form the marble statue assumes out of the endless possible shapes. In this case the formal cause shapes the marble statue. It is technically called an *accidental form* if it gives shape to a body that already exists. The accidental form affects a body without changing its concrete substance or the type of being it is.

A formal cause need not limit its influence only to the shape assumed by a material body. By actuating the matter itself from within, it also determines the type of material being that is to result from a natural process of change. In this case it is called *substantial form*. It makes the matter *be* wood or a dog, etc. The internal organization, structure, proportion and fundamental characteristics of bodies differ because of their specifically different *substantial forms*, e.g. wood, gold, oxygen and dog, etc. Still they are all equally bodies or material beings but they are of different types due to different *substantial forms*.

Though we speak of *matter* and *form* as distinct principles of being they should not be thought of as things capable of separate existence. No matter can exist unless it is of a specific type, i.e. unless it is *informed*. Real gold cannot exist unless it is a material object. The same applies to all material forms: they cannot exist unless they are embodied. It is the concrete individual body that is the true subject of existence and whose being is explained in terms of the real principles of matter and form, also called *prime matter* and *substantial form*. In living bodies, the *substantial form* is also commonly referred to by Aristotle as the *soul* or *principle of life*. The type of life determines the specific type of being. A plant is said to have a vegetative life-principle or soul, an animal a sensitive soul and a human being a rational soul.

Individual bodies exist with their specific nature precisely because their matter is actuated and determined by particular formal causes or forms. At the same time, on account of their material principle, bodies have the potential to become different types of material being through a process of change. In this respect there are various degrees of potency to actual existence for any given individual bodies. Thus hydrogen and oxygen are in more immediate potency to become water (H_2O) than sulphuric acid (H_2SO_4) by means of the appropriate chemical changes. Within an individual body, *matter* and *form* are related to each other as *potency* to *actuality*, while constituting a single existent being or ontological individual. This led Aristotle to comment that matter and form are one in a specific concrete individual body:

> ...the proximate matter and the form are one and the same thing, the one potentially, and the other actually ... for each thing is a unity, and the potential and the actual are somehow one.[3]

This is true, notwithstanding the special characteristics of each of the four causes that influence the real existence and unity of an individual body. Because of the pre-eminence of the causal influence of the form within a body we can even speak of identifying the *essence* or *nature* of a thing with its *form*.

Furthermore, we can say that the final cause and the formal cause are one whenever a natural process of change ceases, giving rise to a new type of being or beings, whose form emerges from the potentiality of the matter of the body or bodies involved. Once the forms of bodies are unable to survive, they are reduced to the potentiality of matter.[4] At the same time this enables a new form or forms to emerge from matter to inform or actuate anew the same matter, thereby constituting one or more new individual bodies. The constancy of the end-product of a process of change enables the final and formal causes to be viewed as one upon the completion of the formation of the new individual body or bodies. Hydrogen and oxygen always react to produce water and vice versa. The meaning or purpose of their interaction is the production of water through the actual emergence of this form from its potential state in the matter of hydrogen and oxygen.

Summary

To understand a real concrete body, we need to realize that it is an *actually existing* individual material being whose form (*formal cause*) makes its matter (*material cause*) the specifically determined type of being that it is, thereby achieving the purpose of its existence (*final cause*). An external agent (*efficient cause*), by its action on the matter of a previously existing body or bodies, is responsible for bringing this individual body into being with its specific character or nature (*form*). Any individual body is capable of changing into some other specifically different type of individual body or bodies. This means the matter of any body is *in potency to become* something specifically different from what it *actually is* when it is subjected to the causal influence of a suitable efficient causal agent that is capable of drawing out or inducing one or more new forms from within its matter. In this way, something material always exists, but the concrete subject of existence, what actually exists, may change from time to time. What is *actually* one thing *is also potentially* something different.

3   Aristotle's biology of human reproduction

Aristotle, working within his metaphysical conceptual framework, set about explaining the reproduction or generation of animals in general, and of humans in particular. He observed that the usual monthly menstrual flow of blood ceased when a woman became pregnant. He furthermore observed that a woman did not become pregnant unless a man had sexual intercourse with her, thereby depositing some semen in her vagina. These were the facts at his disposal, without any knowledge of the cell theory, the existence of ova or of spermatozoa. He knew there must be an efficient cause or an active agent to start the generative process. He likewise knew there must be some suitable material for the active agent to work on to form a specific offspring instead of a generic mammal. It is clear that the model of the sculptor with the block of marble or of the potter with a supply of clay was uppermost in his mind. He assumed the woman's role was passive, supplying her blood as the material needed for forming the offspring. The male provided the formative activity that was to change her blood into a living offspring:

> For there must needs be that which generates and that from which it generates; ... If, then, the male stands for the effective and active, and the female, considered as female, for the passive, it follows that what the female would contribute to the semen of the male would not be semen but material for the semen to work upon. This is just what we find to be the case, for the catamenia have in their nature an affinity to the primitive matter.[5]

It is clear that Aristotle did not think the woman did any more than provide the material for the male agent to work on, somewhat like clay being fashioned into a jar by the potter. The whole material constitution of the offspring is derived from the mother, while the father's semen actively induces the form, i.e. the specific live character.[6] This means that the offspring is only derived from the male as '...that which imparts the motion and as the form'.[7] The father '...only makes a living creature by the power which resides in the semen...'.[8] Aristotle even goes further saying: 'Nature uses the semen as a tool and as possessing motion in actuality....'[9] In other words, the male semen has an active power that moves and changes the mother's blood, shaping it from within into a living young offspring. Of course, the matter in this case is already highly specialized. According to Aristotle the human female menstrual blood has the potency to become all the parts of the human body once it is acted upon by the specific heat and vital power of the semen's πνεῦμα which may be translated as air, breath, wind, spiritus or better transcribed as *pneuma*. In this way the menstrual blood becomes alive with a vegetative soul or form from the time of conception.[10]

When the semen mixes with the menstrual blood a κυήμα (kuēma) is formed, translated as 'embryo' and defined by Aristotle as '...the first mixture of male and female'.[11] He compares the action of rennet coagulating milk to that of the semen on the menstrual blood, causing it to set over a period of several days. This constitutes an embryo that could be compared to a true seed or even an egg.[12] It is with ingenious insight that Aristotle compares the early embryo to the seed of a plant that grows when planted in the soil. The seed does not become a plant before it sprouts and grows. The mother's womb would be the 'soil' and the blood would be the nourishment provided to sustain the embryo once it had exhausted its own energy supplies.[13]

The 'solidifying' of the menstrual blood by means of the action of the semen enables the woman to conceive, i.e. to receive and hold within herself the embryo that has been formed instead of the whole mixture being lost. In Aristotle's words:

> If the seed remain within for seven days then it is certain that conception has taken place; for it is during this period that what is known as effluxion takes place.[14]

He specifies up to seven days for conception following the setting of the menstrual blood mixed with the semen. Though the blood is not considered to be itself a living being in actuality, it is certainly one in potency. By being set as a result of the action of the semen, the blood would have been formed into a living being by the end of the first week, by which time conception would have taken place. The following words of Aristotle certainly confirm this impression:

> What is called effluxion is a destruction of the embryo within the first week, while abortion occurs up to the fortieth day; and the greater number of such embryos as perish do so within the space of forty days.[15]

He takes for granted that the mass of blood is formed into a single living being from the outset. Even with twins this is the case since there is a definite range of proportions of blood to semen required for the constitution of an embryo to occur. Twins are only formed if there is sufficient semen in excess of the normal amount to match a similar excess of supply of menstrual blood.[16] For Aristotle, conception refers to the woman's receiving and holding on to an individual embryo formed out of the mass of homogeneous blood. It never occurred to him to think that a single embryo might divide to give origin to identical twins. Much less could he have entertained the possibility that two or more early embryos might aggregate to form one definitive embryo.

He continues his description of what occurs in a general way, without wishing to make it too precise, in the following terms:

> In the case of male children the first movement usually occurs on

the right-hand side of the womb and about the fortieth day but if the child be a female then on the left-hand side and about the ninetieth day. These and suchlike phenomena are usually subject to differences that may be summed up as differences of degree.

About this period the embryo begins to resolve into distinct parts, it having hitherto consisted of a fleshlike substance without distinction of parts....

In the case of a male embryo aborted about the fortieth day, ... the embryo is revealed as big as one of the large kind of ants; and all the limbs are plain to see, including the penis, and the eyes also, which as in other animals are of great size. But the female embryo, if it suffers abortion during the first three months, is as a rule found to be undifferentiated; if however it reach the fourth month it comes to be subdivided and quickly attains further differentiation.[17]

He links quickening and differentiation into distinct parts at 40 days for the male and 90 days for the female. This is the reason why traditionally he has been interpreted as placing the beginning of the individual boy and girl at those times respectively. This is the origin of the period of 40 days after which the abortion of a fetus would be regarded morally as the equivalent of homicide.

We know Aristotle was mistaken in his account of the formation of the male after 40 days and the female after 90 days. By day 53 the external genitalia still appear to be sexless (See Appendix III). It has been suggested that he probably mistook the remainder of the tail fold at day 40 for the penis. All normal embryos would have appeared in this way to be male, while those that were developing abnormally and did not show any part of the tail fold would have been considered to be female. In fact, it should be noted that a large proportion of embryos that are abnormal appear to be undifferentiated and are usually spontaneously aborted. By day 90 the genitalia are quite apparent. This is one plausible explanation for Aristotle's view that boys are formed after 40 days and girls after 90 days.[18]

4   Aristotle's philosophical theory of human reproduction

It is now necessary to ask why Aristotle adopted his position on the origin of the individual human offspring. His starting point, as we have seen, is his idea of the male being the active principle – the efficient cause – while the female provides only the material as a potential and passive contribution to the offspring's formation. He is also convinced that '...what already exists potentially is brought into being only by what exists actually'.[19] This means that the male is the efficient cause of the offspring, thereby explaining his privileged status in the process of procreation. This need not be done directly as Aristotle does admit the sufficiency of a series of subordinated causes. He illustrates this with reference to a chain of 'automatic machines' where one moves another, which provides an example of the necessary contact between the efficient cause (male) and the effect (offspring).[20]

In practice, the male parent's soul's desire provides the semen that is the bearer of the *pneuma*, which is always the instrument of soul be it in the male, the embryo, or the semen, or even water.[21] The *pneuma* is the active agent that induces movement or change in the menstrual blood without any physical part of the semen becoming part of the embryo itself. An internal principle of life is actualized within the newly constituted embryo to control maintenance, growth and development as an orderly work of the embryo's own nature.[22] Heat and cold certainly play their part in the causal process but they cannot account for the rationale of the formal cause in the *pneuma* that regulates the specific type of conception and its subsequent development. This also depends on the specific potential of the female material (i.e. menstrual blood) for a specific semen's *pneuma* to induce life-giving form by its characteristic movement.[23] Hence a man and a woman can generate only human offspring, not sheep. All things considered, including visual inspections, Aristotle concludes about a week is needed to solidify the menstrual blood to form an embryo. A new live form arises through the causal influence of the semen and its *pneuma's* characteristic life-giving movements, thereby enabling a conception to occur and a pregnancy to begin.

Aristotle presses the analogy of the embryo to a seed sown in the ground whose parts are undifferentiated and in a state of potency until the first principle of growth becomes distinct when a shoot is put forth to provide nourishment.[24] The heart in Aristotle's view is the corresponding first principle for the embryo and is the instrument or organ of the nutritive soul once the embryo is constituted into an individual living being. From the start, it is the principle of nourishment and growth of the living individual. Once it is an actual individual living being it must be nourished in order to grow. The reverse is also true: once something is nourished and grows as a whole, a living individual being must be formed. The formative action of the *pneuma* during the first week is to achieve this stage of unity and actuality of the individual organism. This enables the nourishment and growth of the individual being as a whole to take place.[25]

We must understand that for Aristotle the heart is essentially a nutritive organ since it concocts and distributes blood, the source of nourishment both for self-maintenance and for growth:

> For everywhere the nutriment may be divided into two kinds, the first and the second; the former is 'nutritious', being that which gives its essence both to the whole and to the parts; the latter is concerned with growth, being that which causes quantitative increase.[26]

As such this is a faculty or power that is common to plants and animals:

> ...(for this nutritive power exists in all alike, whether animals or plants, and this is the same as the power that enables an animal or plant to generate another like itself, that being the function of them all if naturally perfect).[27]

Here we find Aristotle indicating that generation itself is akin to the nutritive faculty in as much as generation of offspring is produced from the menstrual blood through the power of the semen, both of which are concocted from life sustaining blood. The semen is a very highly concocted residue derived from blood. Hence we must not be surprised to find Aristotle requiring a nutritive or vegetative soul for the early embryo to survive and function. The next question is whether he requires anything beyond a nutritive soul to explain the existence and activities of the early human embryo.

It is clear that Aristotle believes that it suffices to hold that the embryo, once constituted, is endowed only with a nutritive soul. He can find no evidence of any activity other than nutrition in the early embryo. Plainly this can be explained by a nutritive soul alone. He states his position quite clearly:

> It is plain that the semen and the unfertilized embryo, while still separate from each other, must be assumed to have the nutritive soul potentially, but not actually, except that ... it absorbs nourishment and performs the function of the nutritive soul. For at first all such embryos seem to live the life of a plant. And it is clear that we must be guided by this in speaking of the sensitive and the rational soul. For all three kinds of soul, not only the nutritive, must be possessed potentially before they are possessed in actuality.[28]

To be assured of the actual presence of the 'nutritive soul' it is not enough for the mother alone to draw nourishment: this must also be done by the newly formed embryo for itself. It suffices to show that a new individual living being is present when a new individual begins to be nourished as a whole. This is the typical activity of the nutritive soul. The same principle applies to discern the presence of the sensitive soul in actuality. Just as the heart is the first principle of the nutritive soul in action, the simplest organ of the sense of touch would be the relevant first principle of any of an animal's senses to experience a sensation. The following passage of Aristotle speaks for itself:

> Plainly those principles whose activity is bodily cannot exist without a body, e.g. walking cannot exist without feet.[29]

It is quite clear that '...an animal must have sensation'[30], and consequently must have acquired whatever is necessary for any particular sense to have a sensation, especially the sense of touch. Aristotle obviously assumes:

> ...without a sense of touch it is impossible to have any other sensation; for everybody possessing soul has the faculty of touch....[31]

The early embryo for Aristotle could not yet be an animal in actuality but only a potential animal[32] because he assumes:

> ...if it is necessary that the animal should have sensation and if it is then first an animal when it has acquired sensation, we ought to consider the original condition to be not sleep but only something resembling sleep, such a condition as we find also in plants, for indeed at this time animals do actually live the life of a plant.[33]

He applies the same line of reasoning for an animal to have some minimal sort of knowledge:

> But the function of an animal is not only to generate (which is common to all living things), but they all of them participate also in a kind of knowledge, some more and some less, and some very little indeed. For they have sense-perception, and this is a kind of knowledge.[34]

Here Aristotle distinguishes degrees of sense activity, i.e. ranging from the bare minimum in the sensations of touch and their accompanying sense-perceptions to fine perceptions by the other four sense organs. The fact that some minimum sensation of touch is shared by all animals may have led him to believe there is some common stage of development shared by all animals before they differentiate into specific particular types of animal.

In other words, during the development of an embryo it would become an animal in general without yet being a particular type, say a horse or a dog or even a man. The final stage of development into a particular animal or man would only be reached after the various sense organs had differentiated and become distinct. No doubt the apparent similarities in appearance of all early embryos would have been interpreted as support for this view, granted his lack of knowledge of the cell theory and modern organogenesis. As the forms of horse, cow, dog and man are very different and distinct, he could not accept that these various species are actually formed until their bodily appearance could provide grounds to support such a belief. Hence he postulated this 'generic animal' stage between the possession of the vegetative soul and that of the specific animal or man. Naturally, quite some time is required for all this to happen – in fact 40 days are indicated.

He concludes that the gradual formation of a human individual requires a true succession of souls, involving the corruption (departure) of one soul (= form) followed by the generation of another in the same matter. When the embryo is first formed it would have a nutritive or vegetative soul. When this disappears in due time it would be replaced by the sensitive soul as a result of the causal influence of the specific semen's *pneuma*. Finally, in the case of a human, the rational soul would appear at some time, not specified by Aristotle, from outside matter in a mysterious way, as though it were divine, to complete the generation of a human offspring.[35] This is required by Aristotle because the soul does not use a physical organ for reasoning in the way that seeing requires an eye. A functioning brain is recognized as a pre-condition for thought, but is not the organ of thought itself.

In this sense, the rational soul is regarded as non-material, even though it is one with matter to form a human being. The formative process appears to be totally subordinated to realizing its final cause, i.e. reproducing another of the kind that started the generative process in the first place. It ceases its causal influence only when the specific animal or human individual is completely formed. This is how he himself puts it:

> As they develop they also acquire the sensitive soul in virtue of which an animal is an animal. For, e.g. an animal does not become at the same time an animal and a man or a horse or any other particular animal. For the end is developed last, and the

peculiar character of the species is the end of the generation in each individual. Hence arises a question of the greatest difficulty, which we must strive to solve to the best of our ability and as far as possible. When and how and whence is a share in reason acquired by those animals that participate in this principle? ... It remains, then, for the reason alone so to enter [i.e. from outside] and alone to be divine, for no bodily activity has any connection with the activity of reason.[36]

One cannot but help feel the influence of the 'potter and clay' model of efficient causality here. At first the clay is a solid mass, then a vague vessel shape before it finally assumes, under the moulding influence of the potter's expert hands, its final shape to become a vase in actuality. He felt justified in all this because he could find no evidence to show the presence of activities requiring a sensitive soul in the very early stages of life of the embryo after its conception.

Aristotle is well aware that all the parts of the future animal are potentially present in the menstrual blood.[37] All the same the special movements of the male semen's *pneuma*, acting as the instrument of the male parent, are required for these same parts to be actuated or formed. Furthermore, this is done successively in order to give rise to the nutritive and sensitive souls in actuality:

> The agency by which the parts of animals are differentiated is air, not however that of the mother nor yet of the embryo itself as some of the physicists say.[38]

He further explains the relationship of the power of the nutritive soul to matter:

> For the material by which this latter grows is the same as that from which it is constituted at first; consequently also the power which acts upon it is identical with that which originally gener-ated it; if then this acting power is the nutritive soul, this is also the generative soul, and this is the nature of every organism, existing in all animals and plants.[39]

Of course, this does not commit him to any preformationist embryology whereby all the parts of the embryo, from the start, exist in miniature. If this were so, the processes of differentiation and development would be reduced to growth alone and what already existed completely preformed in actuality would simply grow bigger in size.

Aristotle, on the contrary, supports the theory of epigenesis, i.e. the formation and actualization of new parts that formerly existed only potentially. New parts and organs do come into actual existence. However, we must bear in mind that the degree of potentiality of the various parts in the female material, and in the embryo immediately after its constitution, is quite close to actualization. In short, the early embryo, in Aristotle's view, does not actually possess sense organs, but it has the potency to enable them to be formed and developed in due time under the formative influence of the causal actions of the external agent, the *pneuma* of the male semen. Epigenesis need not necessarily exclude all trace of preformationism. The gradual formation of all the parts and organs of the adult animal could already be predetermined by the specific constitution of a particular embryo. If this were the case the undifferentiated parts could very well exist in the embryo in varying degrees of potency to actualization.[40]

In the Aristotelian way of thinking, humans generate humans, thereby reproducing themselves. The efficient and the final causes of the process are essentially the same. The natural process of generation and reproduction does not cease until it achieves its purpose.[41] The germ or seed determines the formation of a specific offspring but in turn is itself the fruit of the same kind of living creature.[42] Once the embryo is formed and is acted upon by the *pneuma* of the semen it gradually and successively becomes in actuality what it already is in potency. As he succinctly puts it:

> ...when we are dealing with definite and ordered products of Nature, we must not say each *is* of a certain quality because it *becomes* so, but rather that they *become* so and so because they *are* so and so, for the process of Becoming or development attends upon Being and is for the sake of Being, not *vice versa*.[43]

Because man has a nutritive, sensitive and rational soul, and because it does not appear how these could come into actual existence all at once in natural human generation, Aristotle thinks it is necessary that there be successive generations, i.e. that the sensitive soul appear later than the nutritive soul. It would also seem that Aristotle requires the actual presence of sense organs, at least in their minimal structures, as a precondition for the presence of sensitive soul:

> Thus we should say, because man is an animal with such and such characters, therefore is the process of his development necessarily such as it is; and therefore is it accomplished in such and such an order, this part being formed first, that next, and so on in succession;....[44]

Finally, one would not be surprised to find Aristotle requiring a certain size or amount of matter for the presence of various types of natural bodies. Successive stages for the presence of organs would then depend, in part, on the achievement of the requisite size:

> ...of all things naturally composed there is a limit or proportion of size and growth; this is due to the soul, not to fire, and to the essential formula rather than to matter.[45]

This would also mean that a certain minimum mass of material would be needed to constitute a living being, be it vegetative with a nutritive soul or animal with a specific sensitive soul (e.g. that of a horse).

Unlike Plato, Aristotle conceives of the soul in man as the form of the body, the life-principle that enables matter to become a man in actuality.[46] He makes his point quite explicitly:

> If one is to find a definition which will apply to every soul, it will be 'the first actuality of a natural body possessed of organs'.[47]

There is no doubt that Aristotle requires some minimal, but actual, formation of sense organs for the presence of a sensitive soul and the complete generation of a specific animal. This would also be required in the case of a human, irrespective of the precise moment of animation by the rational soul – an issue he never explicitly resolved. This position, however, does not commit Aristotle to the view that a particular animal or man must always be actually exercising the faculty of sensation through its organs. He merely requires the actual possession of the acquired capacity ready for use in experiencing some form of sensation, not the actual experience of sensations. He illustrates this by reference to sleeping and waking states.[48] One who sleeps retains the active capacity to enjoy sensations even though they may not be experienced during sleep. A sensitive soul is required for both waking and sleeping. The same applies to a rational soul that enables a man to have rational self-conscious knowledge. One does not cease to be a man during sleep.

He takes the unity of soul (form) and the living body further still:

> The soul is the cause and first principle of the living body.[49]

This means that the soul ultimately accounts for all that the living body is, namely, something really existent, corporeal, living, vegetative, animal and, finally, human. This is quite significant, since for Aristotle, the efficient, formal and final causes are closely inter-related in the generation of animals and humans. The process ceases only when the appropriate specific form is present, actuating the matter to be an essentially complete specific living animal or human individual. The whole living body is a natural expression of the soul. As Aristotle puts it:

> ...all natural bodies are instruments of the soul; and just as is the case with the bodies of animals, so with those of plants. This shows that they exist for the sake of the soul.[50]

It is ever necessary to be on guard not to interpret *soul* in such a context in any other sense than the form or actuality of matter organized into a living organism whose parts, organs and functions are for the benefit of the totality of what is alive. There is no room for a Platonic or Cartesian dualistic concept of a soul that is not one with the living body, its life-principle, in Aristotle's anthropology.

Summary

For Aristotle, then, the male is the efficient cause of human generation through the *pneuma* of the semen. This causes the menstrual blood to set within a week when conception occurs, and whereby a vegetative or nutritive soul is acquired as life begins. The *pneuma* continues its causal activity, enabling differentiation and development to take place while growth continues. When the basic organs required for sensation are formed, the sensitive soul arises by about the fortieth day, thereby enabling the embryo, by now a fetus, to begin to enjoy animal life. Subsequently, by some mysterious divine intervention the rational soul appears from outside and makes the living body a human being enjoying vegetative, sensitive and rational life. This is the gist of Aristotle's account and it remained unchallenged for about two thousand years.

5   Aristotle's heritage and its unanswered questions

We might smile at some of Aristotle's theories and conclusions. The fact remains that he dominated the scene for about two thousand years. We must not judge his great achievements by criteria derived from our scientific discoveries and methods of observation. The birth of science followed an extremely long and laborious gestation on the part of humanity. Aristotle's teachings held sway all during that period because nobody was able to successfully challenge his positions with any reasonable degree of popular support until the eighteenth century. The accuracy of his common-sense observations, his astute guesses, his penetrating philosophical insights and analyses and the power of his logical reasoning have all guaranteed that both his accomplishments and his errors have had a determining influence in the shaping of the language and conceptions of our Western culture in relation to human procreation.

Aristotle's most serious handicap was his complete lack of factual biological knowledge of the existence and functions of the ovum and the spermatozoon. We cannot blame him for having recourse to the menstrual blood in the circumstances. It would have been difficult in those times to imagine how the blood might have played an active role in generation together with the male semen. His solution was to reduce the female contribution in the generation of offspring to simply one of providing passive material that was to be shaped by the activity of the *pneuma* in the male semen. Might it not have been just as plausible to concede an active role for the female contribution as to postulate the existence of the *pneuma* in the semen acting as an instrument of the male?

It was this biological error, I believe that led him into the *potter and clay* model of causality with the male being considered the efficient cause through the *pneuma* of the semen, as well as being the final cause from the beginning to the end of the process. The *pneuma*, by means of its life-bearing movements, was thought to give rise to the form or soul in the blood once it had been solidified through the semen's action and given rise to a conception. Having uncritically taken for granted that the female material was purely passive, the *pneuma* had to be regarded as an external agent gradually working on the blood. Hence the need for a succession of souls corresponding to the various stages of formation that had to be reached. This would have reflected the making of a clay vase by a potter.

Granted a week for the initial conception, was it really necessary to require first a nutritive soul, followed by the sensitive soul when the sense organs had become distinct? He did not allow for the possibility of the original embryo's active potency to develop sense organs. In this way a sensitive soul could have informed the embryo from the outset of conception. Could not the embryo's sensitive soul begin functioning at the nutritive level while its sensitive activities were in a potential state until the sense organs became distinct through the processes of differentiation and growth? He should have admitted the possible presence of something active in the embryo that would both condition and influence the further shaping of sense organs by its action and at the same time constitute their existence in potency in the embryo, already informed by a sensitive soul. After all, human semen's *pneuma* could only fashion a human individual from an embryo conceived by a woman, not by a cow. The embryo must be oriented to develop in a specific way from the beginning.

Once it is conceded the human embryo is an individual living creature (and Aristotle never questions this) would this not suffice to be a true human individual with the potential for developing sense organs? Was it necessary to require the actual experience of some sensations to be constituted into a human being? Was he too much influenced by how the embryo and fetus looked during visual inspections in determining the requisite minimum bodily formation of the embryo for the presence of the sensitive soul? Though he did not actually say when the rational soul informs the fetus, surely it must have been by the time of birth or at least a few months afterwards. Yet such an infant would only possess the potential to exercise rational functions, not an actually acquired capacity ready for use.

If he had allowed for an active role for the female genetic material, in addition to the male semen, he would have been able to contemplate other possibilities. Would it not have been possible for a single living being to result from the interaction and eventual fusion of both active genetic contributions? Could not this living being be animated by a single life-principle that would enable the embryo to begin to draw nourishment in actuality whilst its sensitive organs and activities would still exist only potentially? As a single life-principle, or soul, performs nutritive and sensitive activities in the animal, could this same life-principle not be present from the very constitution of the embryo, regulating the development and growth of both nutritive and sensitive organs? Though the activities of nourishment and sensation are different, does this exclude the possibility of the same single life-principle (soul) beginning to function first with nutritive functions and subsequently with sensitive activities after the appropriate sense organs had developed?

In the adult animal, we do not have both functions always in operation: is it essential for both to function from the outset in actuality, provided there is a single live embryo present? Could the same logic be applied to the presence of the rational soul from the first constitution of the human embryo? In this case could it not be already a human individual whose rational soul is only actually functioning at the nutritive level, but still having the potential to experience sensations and perform rational acts when organic development is more progressed? Was it really necessary to invent *pneuma* in a theory of causality that gives pre-eminence to men at the expense of women in the generation of human offspring?

While we cannot really blame Aristotle for not asking these questions, we should ask them. We should attempt to seek answers to them in the light of all the biological evidence available in our own day and the philosophical insights presently at our disposal. We are dealing with questions whose traditional answers were quite false and uncritically accepted as true for almost two thousand years. It is time to carefully review all the factors pertaining to these questions and try to arrive at some answers by means of critical reflection on the relevant scientific facts.

6   Aristotle's influence on Aquinas and Christendom

Aristotle's views on human reproduction acquired great historical weight in Christian Europe on account of their substantial adoption by the outstanding philosopher and theologian St Thomas Aquinas (d.1274). It is true to say that Aristotle's general views on the origin of the individual human being held sway from prior to Christian times right through to the Middle Ages and beyond for several centuries.

In one of his earliest writings, commenting on the *Book of Sentences* of Peter Lombard where the conception of Jesus Christ was being discussed, Aquinas states that Christ was conceived instantly by the divine power of the Holy Spirit. This is so, he argues, because his conception, unlike that of others, should not precede the completion of the formation of his natural flesh. This means that *he* was conceived at the same time that conception occurred. Simultaneously the blood was changed to *his* body, organs were formed, ensoulment took place and the animated body was assumed by the Divine Person. Making a reference to St Augustine (d.430) who expressed a similar opinion in his letter to St Jerome (d.420), Aquinas maintains the view that in all other cases the conception of the male child is not completed until the fortieth day, while that of the female child lasts until the ninetieth day.[51] With few exceptions, Aquinas adheres to the views of Aristotle almost to the letter. This is indicative of the little progress made in biology and scientific method during the previous thousand years.

Aquinas' texts are self-explanatory for one who has been introduced to the theories of Aristotle. Here is a typical text that gives a brief summary of his position:

> In the higher animals brought into being through coitus, the active power resides in the male's semen, as Aristotle says (*cf. G.A.* 740b, 24) while the material of the foetus is provided by the female. The vegetative life-principle exists in this material right from the beginning, not in its secondary state of actuality but in its primary state of actuality, just as for instance the sense-soul exists in those who are asleep. When, however, it begins to draw upon nourishment then it becomes actually operative. This

matter is then transmuted by a power in the husband's semen until the sense-soul becomes actual in it. It is not as though this force in the semen becomes the sense-soul, for in that case the generator and the generated would be the same, and again, this would be more like nutrition and growth than generation, as Aristotle says (*cf. G.A.* 321a, 22). However, after the sense-soul has been brought into being in the main part of the one generated by the power of the active principle in the semen, then the sense-soul of the offspring begins working towards the enlargement of its own body by nutrition and growth. However, the active power in the semen ceases to exist when the semen dissolves and the vital spirit in it vanishes. There is nothing impossible about this since this force is not the principal agency but the instrumental one, and the activity of an instrumental cause always ceases once the effect has been produced.[52]

Aquinas drives home the point very clearly that the vital functions of the embryo are derived from its own soul, not that of the mother, nor from the formative power present in the semen:

...vital functions such as feelings, nutrition and growth cannot be derived from an external source. Thus it must be said that the nutritive life-principle [*anima*, soul] pre-exists in the embryo from the beginning, then the sense-soul and finally the intellective soul.[53]

In the following passage Aquinas shows that there is a succession of generations, in which the more perfect souls include the powers and functions of the lower forms or souls. He goes beyond Aristotle by clearly stating that the intellective or rational soul is created by God at the completion of the human reproductive process to give origin to a human being:

We must say then that, since the coming into existence of a being involves the dissolution of another being, it must be held that, both in the case of men and of other animals, when a more perfect form supervenes this brings about the dissolution of the preceding one. However, it does so in such a way that the second form possesses whatever the first one does and something more into the bargain. And thus in man, as in the other animals, the final substantial form comes about through many comings-into-being and dissolutions. This is apparent in the case of animals brought into being by the process of putrefaction. Therefore it must be said that the intellective soul is created by God at the completion of man's coming-into-being. This soul is at one and the same time both a sensitive and nutritive life-principle, the preceding forms having been dissolved.[54]

Aquinas seems to emphasize the unity of the soul and the body more than Aristotle. It is the one soul that accounts for the corporeal, vegetative, organic, sensitive and rational dimensions of the human being. He continues:

Aristotle is not saying merely that the soul actuates a body, but that it is the activating part of an organic physical body that has the power to live, and that such power does not exist apart from the soul.... And so it is said that the soul is the actuation of a body and so on, meaning that due to the soul it is a body, and is organic and has power to live. But the first actuation has a relation of potentiality to the second, which we call activity; and there is no such potentiality apart from or excluding the soul.[55]

This last sentence means that the soul is not only needed for the range of all human activities when they are actually being employed, but also to confer the active capacity to do so when one is not actually exercising some of them, say when one is asleep, drugged or in a coma.

As can easily be seen, Aquinas follows Aristotle in this area with a few significant differences. One such is his account of the creation by God of the intellective soul within the embryo after 40 and 90 days for males and females respectively. He also alters the notion of conception to include rational animation in addition to the initial conception or formation of the body from the menstrual blood. His expanded notion of complete conception now covers the entire process from the imparting of the vegetative soul right through to the acquisition of a sensitive soul and rational ensoulment when a human being is truly constituted. This broader notion of complete conception spans successive generations of living beings until the final stage of the formation of the body and the development of the essential sense organs is achieved 40 days after intercourse.

Conception may now refer to the initial formation of the body or the more perfect formation of the body of the human individual required for sensitive and rational ensoulment. A human being cannot be said to be conceived in the complete sense, according to Aquinas, before actually coming into personal existence through animation by an intellective soul. It is possible to employ both meanings of *conceive* and say: '*I* began to be when *I* was conceived', as well as saying: '*I* did not exist when my mother conceived.' In this latter case one would be using the term in the Aristotelian sense of imparting the nutritive soul and retaining the blood that is *set* in the womb within seven days of intercourse. In the former case the term would be used in Aquinas' sense to refer to the complete formation of an embryonic human being. At times Aquinas does use *conceive* in the Aristotelian sense of *flesh being conceived* before rational ensoulment takes place.[56]

Conceive, when used in the active voice, may have two meanings in the Aristotelian theory of human reproduction. A woman may be said *to have conceived* a week after sexual intercourse when the vegetative soul informs the menstrual blood once it has set. She may also be said to have conceived a human being 40 days after sexual intercourse by which time sensitive and rational ensoulment are said to have occurred. In either case, the clear meaning is that the woman has succeeded in taking the first step towards becoming pregnant and giving birth to a child.

Conceive may be used passively in the Aristotelian sense to refer to the fruit of the original active conception, when the embryo is conceived with a vegetative soul only. There is also a second passive meaning of *conceive* when it is used of a personal subject, to refer to the complete formation of, and hence the beginning of, an embryonic human being. Hence one could say: 'My mother might not have known, but God knew when *I* was conceived.' In the normal way of speaking we usually link the active and passive meanings of the term *conceive* when we simply say: '*My mother conceived me in winter*', without any reference to the length of the process after the act of sexual intercourse. Certainly Aquinas' expanded notion of *conception* is closer to the common-sense point of view.[57] Here is an instance where theological reflection on the conception of Christ could actually have given a pointer in the right direction to human reproductive theory in the pre-scientific age of embryology. It will be necessary later on to try to relate our understanding of conception to contemporary scientific knowledge of human reproduction.

We might also question Aquinas' criteria for settling on Aristotle's 40 days for rational ensoulment. Why not 10, 20 or 30 days? Granted a fetus with an intellective soul cannot exercise rational self-conscious, free or moral acts, we rightly conclude that a fetus lacks the acquired capacity to do so because the brain is not yet sufficiently developed. However, it would have the natural potential to develop and acquire such a capacity ready for immediate employment as occasions arise. Aquinas would have been well aware of this. It is this first actuation of the intellective soul that constitutes a human being just as the first actuation of the sensitive soul makes a living being an animal.

We may question whether a human being need necessarily have acquired the second actuation of the intellective soul which would consist in actually exercising rational activities. Surely a sleeping, drugged or comatose man does not cease to be a man. These are good reasons to believe that once a living individual human embryo is constituted it could, from the outset, be animated with an intellective soul that would be the first actuation or the substantial form of the human body. In this case there would already be an actual human being with the natural potential to develop, in due time, all the organs required for vegetative, sensitive and rational activities.

We must ask are there any convincing reasons to retain Aquinas' theory of succession of souls in human reproduction when we consider that intellective ensoulment could possibly occur at the beginning of the life of the individual human embryo? Need Aquinas have been committed to retaining the Aristotelian active principle of movement residing in the *pneuma* and shaping the embryo for 40 days if intellective ensoulment could have resulted from an act of creation from within, at the start of the individual embryo's existence? The difference between the beginning of the embryo and of the human being in Aquinas' view is the actual development of different organs. How far need the differentiation of organs progress? Is their actual formation really necessary or could they simply be present potentially in the early embryo once it is animated by an intellective soul? Would it not suffice for the embryo to be definitively individualized? These questions, together with the others previously raised for Aristotle, would need to be answered if Aquinas' account of human reproduction is to retain any grounds of credibility.

7   Harvey's refutation of Aristotle's biology of human reproduction

William Harvey (1578–1657) was an eminent anatomist as well as an enthusiastic disciple of Aristotle. He broke new ground by his observations on the reproduction of deer, since no one had previously undertaken a systematic investigation of any kind of developing mammalian fetus. He was convinced that if he was to trace our origins back to our first beginnings his enquiry into human reproduction 'must be begun from its causes, particularly from its material and efficient cause'.[58] From as early as 1616 in his *Anatomical Lectures* he showed his Aristotelian bent:

It is the male in whom resides the formative power, the active principle, the female in whom there is the place and the material. Wherefore the first principle of generation begins in the male and is perfected in the female... The maker seeks his material as the heat of the heavens the earth below.[59]

Harvey's observations on the generation of chicks led him to believe that this provided the key to understanding the generation of humans. The fertilized egg is a conception itself, the fruit of the union of the male and the female, the seed containing the potential offspring. He puts it as follows:

> For in the same manner and rational order that the chick is fashioned and produced from an egg, so does the foetus of viviparous animals come likewise from a pre-existent conception. There is one and the same generation in all of them, and the first beginning of each is either called an egg or at least something analogous to an egg. For an egg is a conception which is put forth from the body and from which the chick is procreated. A conception is an egg remaining in the body until the foetus within it has acquired its just perfection. In other matters they also agree. They are both living rudiments and they are both animals *in potentia* ... For according to Aristotle's opinion, true seed is that which takes its origin from the coition of two animals, and it derives its virtue from both sexes.[60]

In 1633 Harvey observed the deer of King Charles I during their mating season from mid-September and subsequently at regular intervals to mid-November dissected uteri of some fallow does and red deer hinds. He expected to find a mass of menstrual blood, coagulated to form an egg as a result of its mingling with the buck's or stag's semen from rutting time. This would have been the conception, or egg, referred to above. To his great surprise nothing of the sort was found for many weeks after rutting time. The King's keepers, huntsmen and physicians found it difficult to believe that copulation, presumed to have taken place from the start of the rut, had not already caused conception. The Aristotelian theory of conception had assumed this to be an indisputable fact of experience.

Harvey did not seem to be aware that although the red deer stags and fallow bucks start rutting about mid-September, it is not until about mid-October that the hinds and does come into oestrus. This means that ova could not be fertilized as a result of coitus before this time. Little wonder Harvey could not find any sign of conception in September and early October. In fact, he did not discover evidence of conception until mid-

November when the embryo resembled, not an egg-shaped conception that he expected to find, but a clearly visible elongated mucous filament like a spider's thread prior to implantation in the womb.[61]

Harvey was left to draw his own conclusions:

> ...the foetus does not arise from either the male or the female sperm emitted in coitus, nor from both of them mixed together, as the physicians think, nor from the menstrual blood as being the substance, as Aristotle thought, and that something of the conception is not necessarily made immediately after coitus. And therefore it is not true that in a fertile copulation some material is ready prepared in the uterus, which the power or virtue of the male seed, like a coagulant, should concoct, coagulate and fashion, or reduce into an actual generation, or having dried its outward surfaces enclose in membranes. For nothing is found in the womb for many days.[62]

He furthermore erroneously concluded the ovaries are 'like things utterly unconcerned in generation'.[63] He had not been able to perceive the presence of the ovum or the early embryo because they were too small shortly after intercourse to be seen by the naked eye. In this way he was able to refute the age-old Aristotelian theory of viviparous reproduction for animals and humans alike.

It was not only the absence of a conception and of menstrual blood in the womb, but also the absence of semen that Harvey noticed:

> You will indeed find nothing remaining therein after coitus, for the male sperm either falls out again in a short while or vanishes away, and the blood, having made its circuit, goes back again from the uterus through the vessels.[64]

This was a problem for Harvey as he knew that conceptions of offspring and pregnancies only follow sexual intercourse. If the semen did not remain in the womb, as he thought, then it must be due to some contact made by it that somehow renders the womb fertile. The contact itself had to be life-giving. This suggested the notion of contagion, through which diseases are caught by mere contact. He thought this model might be helpful to explain how reproduction occurs. He did not know of viruses or bacteria. He could only conclude the cause must be incorporeal upon the occasion of the contact of the semen with the womb:

> If, what I have called by the common name contagion, as being derived from spermatic contact in coitus and remaining behind in

the female when the spermatic fluid is no longer present, is the efficient cause and artificer of the future procreation, if, I repeat, this contagion, be it atoms or odour or ferment or any other thing, be unrelated to the nature of a body, then it must needs be a thing incorporeal.[65]

An active power would be exercised by both the female as well as the male in procreation, though Harvey was at a loss to account for the source of this generative power beyond suggesting the Creator, the heavens or the sun:

For it is certain that there is in the egg (as well as in every conception and first rudiment), an operative power which is infused into it not only from the female, but which is also communicated to it first by the male in coitus through his geniture, and that this was first of all given to the male by the heavens or the sun or the Almighty Creator.[66]

Though he could not find any explanation for conception's occurrence, Harvey did have recourse to comparing the conception in the womb with the conception of the soul's thought in the brain. An external object causes the brain to conceive it in some hidden manner through sense-perception. In a similar way the male, through intercourse, mysteriously causes the female's womb to conceive the beginnings of an offspring of the same species or form. As Harvey puts it:

And just as appetite or desire springs from the conception of the brain and this conception in turn from some external object of desire, so also from the male as being the more perfect animal, and as it were, the most natural object of desire, the natural conception arises in the womb of the woman, even as the animal conception is made in the brain.[67]

Harvey shows his Aristotelian roots by reverting to the unity of the final and formal cause to complete his analogy by way of explanation:

The conception, therefore of the egg or of the uterus will be, at least in some manner, similar to the conception of the brain, and the end inheres in both equally in the same way. That is to say, the appearance or form of the chick is in the uterus or egg without any material, just as the concept of his work is in the artificer, as for instance the concept of the house is in the brain of the builder.[68]

Harvey was not entirely satisfied. He could not find any empirical evidence for the design of the future offspring. He knew it must be there somewhere. At least he had disproved Aristotle's view of conception even if he was unable to offer his own biological account to replace it. He knew nothing about chromosomes, genes and DNA molecules. The microscope came too late for him to discover sperm and ovum. Nevertheless, his experiments, observations and discoveries were extremely important in that they first deprived the traditional Aristotelian theory of successive animations in human reproduction of biological support. Harvey himself did not subsequently advance any view on when rational ensoulment occurs or when the individual human being begins. However, his work cleared the way for the philosophical theory of immediate animation or rational ensoulment from the outset to claim some support from the empirical sciences.

8   Decline of Aristotle's theory of human reproduction

Philosophical opinions regarding rational ensoulment did not change much after Aquinas until 1620 when the Flemish physician, Thomas Fienus (Feyens), advanced the view that the semen only requires three days to transform the blood by its coagulating action to prepare it to receive the rational soul.[69] This was indeed a radical challenge to the tradition. He saw no need to postulate any succession of generations or of souls to explain the gradual development of organs and their functions. The rational soul begins to animate the amorphous coagulated mass of blood and give it shape after its infusion on the third day. As Needham puts it:

> ...the soul is the principle which organizes the body from within, arranging an organ for each of its faculties and preparing its own residence, not merely consenting to be breathed into a physical being which has already organized itself. 'The conformation of the foetus is a vital, not a natural, action', he says.[70]

It is important to note that Fienus was arguing against the traditionalists' view from within their own system. He regarded the rational soul as the form of the living body that developed epigenetically from within. He argued that the rational soul was present after birth even though rational functions could not begin to be performed before the age of two or three years. Hence he saw no point in delaying rational animation for some 40 days beyond the conception of the living body that occurs on the third day, even if no evidence of rational functions could be found at that stage. It is the same individual living being that develops continuously from the moment of animation by the rational soul through the entire period of fetal development and gestation up to birth and adulthood.[71]

In the following year, 1621, Paolo Zacchias, a Roman physician, adopted views very similar to those of Fienus, maintaining that the rational soul was infused from the start of conception.[72] He argued that if the rational soul could be actually present after 40 days though its functions were still only in potency, it could likewise be actually present from the start of conception while its functions were in a similar potential state.[73] Zacchias' views gained some support but quite a deal of opposition from the traditionalists. Added weight was given to his thesis on immediate ensoulment in 1644 when Pope Innocent X conferred on him the title of 'General Proto-Physician of the Whole Roman Ecclesiastical State'.[74] Zacchias and Fienus developed their alternative views within the biological and philosophical framework of both Aristotle and Aquinas.

Even though philosophers and theologians were slow to acquaint themselves with the implications of the latest scientific discoveries there was some progress. Professor Short succinctly sums up the situation after Harvey's work:

> In contrast to the Aristotelian view that the 'female testicles' of mammals played no part in reproduction, Niels Stensen of Denmark in 1667 concluded that they contained ova, like the ovaries of birds, and were therefore involved in the reproductive process, and should be called ovaries. Van Leeuwenhoek's discovery of mammalian spermatozoon in 1678, and his suggestion in 1683 that life began when a male spermatozoon impregnated an ovum, set men thinking along the right lines, although it was not until the nineteenth century that fertilization was actually observed.[75]

Though it was only in 1827 that Von Baer discovered and described the female ovum, some philosophers and theologians had gradually come to know of some of the scientific findings of the biologists well before the end of the seventeenth century. It was becoming more difficult, but not impossible, to cling on to the traditional theories of reproduction and the Aristotelian theory of delayed rational animation. Two additional interesting developments gave unexpected support to the theory of immediate rational ensoulment.

The *first* was the biological theory of *preformation* according to which

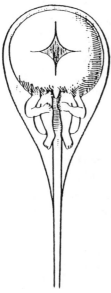

Fig. 2.1. Copy of a seventeenth century drawing by Hartsoeker of a sperm. The miniature human being within it was thought to enlarge after the sperm entered an ovum. From *The Developing Human: Clinically Oriented Embryology*, by K. Moore, Philadelphia: W. B. Saunders, 3rd edn, 1982.

the appearance of different organs and parts in the developing fetus is merely due to the unfolding and growth of parts already differentiated and actually existing in the embryo from the outset. This would be the opposite of the theory of epigenesis which explains the origin of new parts and organs by a process of differentiation, and growth from within the embryo where they previously merely pre-existed potentially.

Two forms of preformation appeared – *ovism* and *animalculism* or *spermism*. *Ovism* held that the female ovum contains the whole of the future organism in a primordial state so that the sperm merely acts as a stimulus to further development and growth. The offspring would be the product of the female egg. *Animalculism* or *spermism* held that the sperm itself already contains a tiny animal (animalcule) or a tiny human being fully formed in miniature (Fig. 2.1). In the case of humans, this was called *homunculus* – a tiny human being that would begin to grow once in contact with the fertile environment of the womb. Needham reports:

> By 1720 the theory of preformation was thoroughly established, not only on the erroneous grounds put forward by Malpighi and Swammerdam, but on the experiments of Andry, Dalenpatius

and Gautier, who all asserted that they had seen exceedingly minute forms of men, with arms, heads and legs complete, inside the spermatozoa under the microscope.[76]

One can imagine how such talk and hazy use of early microscopes would influence the imagination and lend easy support to the theory of immediate animation. If a fully formed human being in miniature was present in the embryo, derived from the egg or the spermatozoon, immediate rational ensoulment would be assumed to have taken place.

The *second* interesting development that helped establish immediate animation was the decline of Aristotelian–Thomistic philosophy among the scholastic philosophers at the time. The *hylomorphic theory* was not always correctly understood. In 1637 Descartes published his *Discourse on Method* in which he proposed his dualistic theory of the human being. He held the soul and body were two distinct substances that formed a union of two realities, but not the unity of a single being. Descartes' own words are quite clear and explicit in his *Discourse on Method:*

> From this I recognised that I was a substance whose whole essence or nature is to be conscious (*de penser*) and whose being requires no place and depends on no material thing. Thus this self (*moi*), that is to say the soul, by which I am what I am, is entirely distinct from the body, and is even more easily known; and even if the body were not there at all, the soul would be just what it is.[77]

His dualism enabled philosophers to think of the soul as present from the start of conception, not as the form of the body, but as a separate reality in close relationship with the body. If the 'self' is thought to be constituted by the soul, it would not matter whether the body united to the soul was tiny and undeveloped. Even when preformationism was discarded, the influence of Descartes' dualism was lasting, along with the theory of immediate rational ensoulment.

The discovery of the active part played by both ovum and spermatozoon in the process of fertilization lent support to the theory of immediate rational ensoulment. Noonan aptly summarizes majority thinking late in the nineteenth century:

> A change in organism was seen to occur at the moment of fertilization which distinguished the resultant from the components. It was easier to mark this new organism off from the living elements which had preceded it than it was to mark it off from some later stage of its organic growth in the uterus. If a moment had to be chosen for ensoulment, no convincing argument now

appeared to support Aristotle or to put ensoulment at a later stage of fetal life.[78]

9   **Revival of Aquinas' version of Aristotle's theory of human reproduction**

Not all who had rejected Aristotle's biology rejected his basic philosophical theory of successive generations of the vegetative, sensitive and rational souls. Joseph Donceel is a vigorous supporter of the theory of delayed rational animation and he cites many authors of the last and present century who think along the same lines in his article published in 1970.[79] He agrees that there is immediate animation from the start of conception, but with a progression from the vegetative to sensitive and to the rational soul. He does not speak of *delayed animation*, but rather of *delayed hominization* because a *Homo*, a human being, is not present prior to rational ensoulment. He firmly believes the human soul is the form of the body, in full agreement with the hylomorphic theory. He holds the organs required for the exercise of rational functions must be already formed if a rational soul is to be present. He does not require that their development be sufficient for the actual exercising of rational functions. Successive souls (forms) are needed because 'to each specific degree of organization there corresponds a soul'.[80] Referring to Aquinas' position, Donceel asserts his own stand too:

> ...it is easy to see that his lack of biological information does not affect his philosophical position. The real reason why he professed delayed hominization was his hylomorphic conception of man. He knew very well that the early embryo was not yet a fully organized human body. In his opinion, this excluded the possession of a real human soul. He was aware that the embryo was virtually, potentially, a human body, that, given a normal development, it would become such a body. But his philosophy prevented him from joining an actual human soul to a virtual human body. If form and matter are strictly complementary, as hylomorphism holds, there can be an actual human soul only in a body endowed with the organs required for the spiritual activities of man. We know that the brain, and especially the cortex, are the main organs of those highest sense activities without which no spiritual activity is possible.[81]

Donceel agrees that the fertilized ovum from the time of fecundation would have a life of its own, that it would be a human organism with its own typically human genetic code, but holds that it would be no more a human being than a live human heart removed from the body of a recently deceased donor during a transplantation operation. He does not admit the presence of 'the virtuality, the power of developing into a human person'[82] suffices to actually constitute a human being. Otherwise, he argues, one would have to admit that each cell of the early embryo would be a person since each cell if separated from the rest during its totipotent stage could, given the right conditions, develop into an identical twin.[83] Donceel himself, after referring to a quotation from Schoonenberg for support,[84] suggests hominization does not occur before several weeks:

> The least we may ask before admitting the presence of a human soul is the availability of these organs: the senses, the nervous system, the brain, and especially the cortex. Since these organs are not ready during early pregnancy, I feel certain that there is no human person until several weeks have elapsed.[85]

Haring, Diamond and Pastrana, in delaying hominization, and with slight variations among themselves, share some ground with the position sustained by Donceel, while K. Rahner admits that the theory of immediate rational ensoulment is open to positive doubt.[86]

Admittedly, most philosophers in the tradition of Aristotle and Aquinas would today still uphold the more recent tradition of immediate rational ensoulment from the time of conception. One weakness in Donceel's position is the unjustified demand for the formation of sense organs and of the brain for rational ensoulment once it is admitted there are no rational functions performed for at least two years. Insufficient reasons seem to be given to justify delaying rational ensoulment after conception and the formation of the individual embryo for some vaguely specified 'several weeks'. He might be right, but his philosophical arguments need to be supported by more solid embryological evidence to determine the minimum period of time after fertilization before which rational ensoulment or hominization could not possibly take place.

10   The Bible and the question of when a human being begins

The Bible has a lot to say about human life but it certainly cannot be used to determine the moment of the origin of the individual human being in the mother's womb. There is the *Genesis* account of the creation of man and woman in the beginning of human history. The message is very positive indeed, in spite of our awareness of personal and collective evil and suffering throughout the ages. Men and women are created in the image and likeness of God. Life is presented as something good – a unique divine gift enabling mankind to be sharers in God's own friendship. In their turn, men and women are invited to communicate that same life to others because it is such a great gift. This remains true even though evil, suffering and death originated in this universe as a result of people abusing their freedom in disobeying God's command. Nevertheless, God promises salvation to all. Much of the Bible is an account of how God realized His plan to save mankind, culminating in the life and death of Jesus Christ.

God's word in the Bible tells people what they must believe and do in order to be saved. The message is couched in the language and culture of the times without necessarily endorsing the scientific presuppositions embedded in the thought patterns and language employed. We should no more look to the Bible for scientific facts of biology or embryology and their philosophical interpretation than for astronomy or paleontology. The Bible is indeed the Book of Life *par excellence*, namely, about the meaning, calling and destiny of human life in God's loving plan of salvation, and about what people must believe and do to be saved. The progress made in understanding the Biblical literary forms in modern exegesis should prevent us repeating the sort of misinterpretations of the Bible made in Galileo's times and beyond. The Bible, correctly interpreted, can never be in conflict with genuine scientific fact. It would be helpful to briefly examine a few passages in the Bible that are sometimes mistakenly claimed to support particular doctrines about when a human individual begins.

Many passages of the Bible refer to human life in the womb, attesting a belief that a caring and loving God is at work forming the human being from the very outset of its constitution, without asserting exactly when, or at what precise stage of embryological development, the individual human being begins to be. A variety of popular beliefs abounded in ancient times.[87] It would be natural for the ancient Jews to express views similar to their contemporaries when they confessed their belief that God was the Lord of life from the very beginning of each person. In the following passage Job is proclaiming his belief in a Provident God, not giving a lesson in embryology:

> Your own hands shaped me, modelled me;
> and would you now have second thoughts, and destroy me?
> You modelled me, remember, as clay is modelled,
> and would you reduce me now to dust?
> Did you not pour me out like milk,

and curdle me then like cheese;
clothe me with skin and flesh,
and weave me of bone and sinew?[88]

A case of resemblance between *Psalm* 104 and an ancient Egyptian hymn
to the sun-god Aton, written by Akhanaton, Amenophis IV about
1400 B.C. is suggested by Needham. The Jews would have been in Egypt
at the time and could have become familiar with its concepts and
terminology, absorbing them into their general culture:

> *Hymn to Aton, the Sun-god who is addressed.*
> Creator of the germ in woman,
> Maker of seed in man,
> Giving life to the son in the body of his mother,
> Soothing him that he may not weep,
> Nurse (even) in the womb.
> Giver of breath to animate every one that he maketh
> When he cometh forth from the womb on the day of his birth.
> Thou openest his mouth in speech,
> Thou suppliest his necessity....[89]

A resemblance to this sort of language is found in other places in the Bible,
in addition to *Psalm* 104: 27–30:

> All creatures depend on you
> to feed them throughout the year;
> you provide the food they eat,
> with generous hand you satisfy their hunger.
> You turn your face away, they suffer,
> you stop their breath, they die
> and revert to dust.
> You give breath, fresh life begins,
> you keep renewing the world.

The Alexandrian Jews sometime during the second century B.C. authored
the *Book of Wisdom* and possibly show signs of some influence of
Aristotelian embryology on their outlook in the following passage
(*Wisdom* 7: 1–4):

> Like all the others, I too am a mortal man,
> descendant of the first being fashioned from the earth,
> I was modelled in flesh within my mother's womb,
> for ten months taking shape in her blood
> by means of virile seed and pleasure, sleep's companion.

> I too, when I was born, drew in the common air,
> I fell on the same ground that bears us all,
> a wail my first sound, as for all the rest.

Here Solomon is showing that he is the same as any other man. The reference is of course to ten lunar months, the equivalent of nine calendar months.

In the *Book of Exodus* 21: 22–23, the law deals with penalties for injuries incurred during a fight. It is interesting to see the provisions for a pregnant woman injured incidentally while men are fighting among themselves. The translation of the Hebrew is as follows:

> If, when men come to blows, they hurt a woman who is pregnant and she suffers a miscarriage, though she does not die of it, the man responsible must pay the compensation demanded of him by the woman's master; he shall hand it over after arbitration. But should she die, you shall give life for life, eye for eye, tooth for tooth, hand for hand, foot for foot, burn for burn, wound for wound, stroke for stroke.

It is to be noted that this text is dealing with unintentional harm done to the pregnant woman. If she dies the penalty is equally grave. If only the fetus dies, a fine is imposed to compensate the loss to the mother and ultimately to the father of a child and future heir. The context of the text is most likely not about the right to life of the fetus, but the damage caused to the parents by such unintentional loss of fetal life.[90] We should not forget that spontaneous miscarriages were as common then as now. They were accepted as a part of life. There was no express prohibition of intentional abortion in the Mosaic Law. This was not needed since the Jews had a very high regard for parenthood and the survival of their race by procreation.[91] Hence this text cannot be used to resolve the question of when a human individual begins.

However, the Greek translation of this same passage in the Septuagint version, made about the year 250 B.C., is somewhat different. This version was made for the Jews living among the Greeks in Alexandria. It was highly authoritative both then and during the early Christian period. It seems the 'perfectly formed' fetus is assumed to be a human being but not when 'imperfectly formed'. The text runs as follows:

> And if two men strive and smite a woman with child, and her child be born imperfectly formed, he shall be forced to pay a penalty: as the woman's husband may lay upon him, he shall pay with a valuation. But if it be perfectly formed, he shall give life for

life, eye for eye, tooth for tooth, hand for hand, foot for foot, burning for burning, wound for wound, stripe for stripe.[92]

The Greek word used for 'be born', here is ἐξέλθῃ (exelthē) which literally means 'comes out'. Possibly there was a conscious effort by the translators to adapt the original text to the situation of their own times in the light of those known stages of fetal development that happened to resemble the Aristotelian account and in view of the injustice of the practice of abortion prevalent among those with whom they lived.[93]

Philo in his first-century reference to this text not only follows the Septuagint version of the *Book of Exodus*, but elaborates on it, giving his reasons for agreeing with it. He regards the formed fetus as a true human being even though quite some time is still required before its birth. We might safely assume that Philo accepts Aristotle's 40-day period as a minimum for the embryo to become a human being. Failing this, perhaps a form that could be recognized as human would suffice.[94] This is how he puts it, adapting the text for his purposes of explaining the moral law forbidding homicide:

> But if any one has a contest with a woman who is pregnant, and strike her a blow on her belly, and she miscarry, if the child which was conceived within her is still unfashioned and unformed, he shall be punished by a fine, both for the assault which he committed and also because he has prevented nature, who was fashioning and preparing that most excellent of all creatures, a human being, from bringing him into existence. But if the child which was conceived had assumed a distinct shape* in all its parts, having received all its proper connective and distinctive qualities, he shall die; for such a creature as that is a man, whom he has slain while still in the workshop of nature, who had not thought it as yet a proper time to produce him to the light, but had kept him like a statue lying in a sculptor's workshop, requiring nothing more than to be released and sent out into the world. *Exodus xxi:22.[95]

This interpretation of Philo could well have made the Aristotelian view more plausible among the early Christians and eventually given support to the theory of delayed rational animation.

We need not be too concerned with *Psalm* 51: 5:

> You know I was born guilty,
> a sinner from the moment of conception.

It is obvious one cannot be a sinner until a human being exists. The meaning of conception here refers to the beginning of the individual human being, whenever that occurs, irrespective of what this term means with reference to the activity of the mother.

Few conclusions can be drawn relevant to our topic from the New Testament account of the virgin birth of Jesus Christ. Luke's purpose in writing about this event, which is as far beyond human comprehension as it is outside the laws of nature, was certainly not to teach anything about when human individuals begin in the natural way. However, Luke's account of the meeting of Mary and Elizabeth is interesting:

> Now as soon as Elizabeth heard Mary's greeting, the child leapt in her womb and Elizabeth was filled with the Holy Spirit. She gave a loud cry and said, ... For the moment your greeting reached my ears, the child in my womb leapt for joy.[96]

To say the least, this text would take for granted that a six-month old fetus is already certainly considered to be a human being by Luke and his contemporaries. This would accord with the common-sense viewpoint on account of its stage of development and its viability to survive outside the mother's womb. This much would have been common knowledge when Luke was writing his Gospel.

This brief review of some of the relevant biblical and related data shows that the Bible does not even ask the question of the moment of the rational ensoulment or the beginning of the individual human being in the womb of the mother. An answer is not given in the Bible and should not be sought there. In other words, the Scriptures do not exempt us from our duty to continue our scientific investigations and philosophical reflections in search of a solution to the pressing question of when each one of us began to be a human individual.

11   The Catholic position on when a human being begins

There would be sufficient interest in knowing the official position of the Catholic Church on the origin of the individual human being to warrant a brief consideration of her teaching on this issue. This interest is shared by both Catholics and non-Catholics alike. One need not believe in the Catholic Church to be interested in her teachings. The fact of the matter is the Catholic Church has never officially taught when the individual human being, endowed with a rational soul, begins in the mother's womb. It would come as no surprise to learn that the Catholic Church's interest in this area is not primarily scientific or philosophical.

Her mission is at the service of the Word of God and the promotion of the Kingdom of Heaven.

From the earliest times the Church has taught the immorality of abortion at any stage after conception. She likewise condemned homicide and sanctioned canonical penalties for it. This naturally led to the question whether every abortion was also homicide or only if performed after a certain stage in the pregnancy. The Catholic Church throughout history has obviously been influenced by the commonly accepted view on the moment of rational ensoulment whenever canonical legislation was being drafted in this regard. This is openly admitted by the Catholic Church:

> It is true that in the Middle Ages, when the opinion was generally held that the spiritual soul was not present until after the first few weeks, a distinction was made in the evaluation of the sin and the gravity of the penal sanctions. In resolving cases, approved authors were more lenient with regard to that early stage than with regard to later stages. But it was never denied at that time that procured abortion, even during the first few days, was objectively a grave sin. This condemnation was in fact unanimous.[97]

In other words the Catholic Church once assumed that the embryo did not become a human being until several weeks after conception. Grisez affirms this remained so in practice until 1869 when Pope Pius IX, in the constitution *Apostolicae Sedis*:

> ...included among those who incur automatic excommunication 'those procuring abortion, if successful', without distinguishing whether the fetus was animated or not. In effect this act endorsed the growing awareness that the old distinction between animated and non-animated fetuses was grounded neither in experimental evidence nor necessary reasons. While this distinction might be maintained theoretically, the arguments of Fienus, Zacchias and others finally had their practical effect.[98]

Once more the Church, in the light of the available biological evidence, made an assumption, except that this time it was in favour of immediate rational ensoulment of the embryo. The 1854 definition of the *Dogma of the Immaculate Conception* of the Virgin Mary herself does not resolve this issue. This means that when Mary began to be as a personal being, she was free of original sin, without determining the precise moment that she was conceived as a human being. This doctrine refers to Mary's sanctification at *her natural conception,* not her mother's act of conceiving.[99] The distinction between the passive and active meanings of conception is quite relevant here.

In a more positive manner the Council of Vienne in 1311–12 defined that it was heretical to:

> hold that the rational or intellectual soul is not in itself and essentially the form of the human body.[100]

The point of this defined doctrine is to clarify and teach that there is no essential dualism in human nature, i.e. that the spiritual soul constitutes one being with the human body so that the soul itself is the life-principle of the body. In this way the unity and integrity of the human being is guaranteed. However, the Council did not specify when this unity of the human being is first constituted.

The Second Vatican Council was quite explicit in what it had to say about the value of life from the beginning, even though it was aware that the question when rational ensoulment took place had not been satisfactorily resolved:

> Life must be protected with the utmost care from conception: abortion and infanticide are abominable crimes.[101]

It is stated more forcefully in the Apostolic See's *Chapter of the Rights of the Family* (23 October 1983) Art. 4:

> Human life must be respected and protected absolutely from the moment of conception.

The benefit of any doubt should go in favour of the embryo from conception.

It was not until 1974, in the context of condemning abortion, that Catholic teaching officially touched on the moment of the origin of the individual human being. This teaching takes for granted the views of the vast majority of ordinary people today that each of us began our lives as individuals at the moment of conception, understood as fertilization. The Church also claimed that modern genetic science supports these views, though she was careful to point out that really this is an issue that should more properly be resolved by philosophers rather than scientists. It is interesting that she did not claim that the moment of the constitution of the individual human being or human person, endowed with a rational soul, is a matter for theology as distinct from philosophy to determine. While she is ever intransigent on the moral issue of deliberate abortion, she did not close the door on the theoretical question of the moment of rational ensoulment and, consequently, on the timing of the constitution of the individual human person.

The relevant texts of the 1974 *Declaration on Procured Abortion* in paragraphs 12 and 13 read as follows:

> 12. In reality respect for human life is called for from the time that the process of generation begins. From the time that the ovum is fertilized, a life is begun which is neither that of the father nor of the mother; it is rather the life of a new human being [= *novi viventis humani*] with his own growth. It would never be made human if it were not human already.
>
> 13. This has always been clear, and discussions about the moment of animation have no bearing on it. Modern genetic science offers clear confirmation. It has demonstrated that from the first instant there is established the programme of what this living being will be: a man, this individual man with his characteristic aspects already well determined. Right from fertilization the adventure of a human life begins, and each of its capacities requires time – a rather lengthy time – to find its place and to be in a position to act. The least that can be said is that present science, in its most evolved state, does not give any substantial support to those who defend abortion. Moreover, it is not up to biological sciences to make a definitive judgment on questions which are properly philosophical and moral, such as the moment when a human person is constituted or the legitimacy of abortion. From a moral point of view this is certain: even if a doubt existed concerning whether the fruit of conception is already a human person, it is objectively a grave sin to dare to risk murder. 'The one who will be a man is already one.'[102]

I have included the Latin words *novi viventis humani* in brackets to show that the true translation there should read 'of a new human living being or creature'. The Church stopped short of categorically asserting that the fertilized egg itself is already a human being or a person. To say that from the first moment of the completion of the process of fertilization the fertilized egg has the genetic programme of a man is not the same as asserting that the fertilized egg itself already is a man (*homo*).

This point is made clearer still by an important footnote to the first sentence of paragraph 13 where it is explicitly stated that the *Declaration* does not intend to resolve the issue of the moment of spiritual or rational ensoulment. Clearly, the living being that the fertilized egg is cannot be a

human being or a person without the spiritual soul, though it can be said
to be *human* life and to have already programmed and predetermined
within itself the genetic individuality or genome of a human individual.
The distinction is important as identical twins are genetically identical and
derive from the same fertilized egg, but they are separate individual
human beings. The text of note 19 in the *Declaration* reads as follows:

> 19. This declaration expressly leaves aside the question of the
> moment when the spiritual soul is infused. There is not a
> unanimous tradition on this point and authors are as yet in
> disagreement. For some it dates from the first instant, for others it
> could not at least precede nidation. It is not within the com-
> petence of science to decide between these views, because the
> existence of an immortal soul is not a question in its field. It is a
> philosophical problem from which our moral affirmation remains
> independent for two reasons: (i) supposing a later animation,
> there is still nothing less than a *human* life, preparing for and
> calling for a soul in which the nature received from parents is
> completed; (ii) on the other hand it suffices that this presence of
> the soul be probable (and one can never prove the contrary) in
> order that the taking of life involve accepting the risk of killing a
> man, not only waiting for, but already in possession of his soul.[103]

Pope John Paul II during his recent visit to Australia rightly said the
following at the Mercy Maternity Hospital, in Melbourne, the Australian
capital of *in vitro* fertilization and research on human embryos.

> In the delicate field of medicine and biotechnology the Catholic
> Church is in no way opposed to progress. Rather, she rejoices at
> every victory over sickness and disability. Her concern is that
> nothing should be done which is against life in the reality of a
> concrete individual existence, no matter how underdeveloped or
> how advanced.[104]

It is interesting to compare this with the words he used earlier in the same
day to about 150 000 people attending a Mass at the Flemington Race
Course, Melbourne: 'Will the Christian community defend the gift of life
from conception to the moment of death?'[105] 'Life in the reality of a
concrete individual existence' seems to be an equivalent alternative
expression to 'from conception to the moment of death'. No reference was
made to the contentious issue of the beginning and end of the presence of
human personhood.

In March 1987 The Congregation for the Doctrine of the Faith of the

Catholic Church issued an *Instruction on Respect for Human Life in its Origin and on the Dignity of Human Procreation – Replies to Certain Questions of the Day*. It did not pretend to:

> ...intervene on the basis of a particular competence in the area of experimental sciences

but rather by way of

> ...expounding the criteria of moral judgement as regards the applications of scientific research and technology, especially in relation to human life and its beginnings.[106]

The Church is well

> ...aware of the current debates concerning the beginning of human life, concerning the individuality of the human being and concerning the identity of the human person.[107]

She accepts the fact that the genetic or biological identity of a new human individual begins at fertilization when a zygote is formed and takes it for granted that this suffices for the presence of a human being, indeed even a personal presence. On the basis of an ordinary human understanding of these facts, the Church adopts a position of prudential certitude in relation to the presence of individual and personal life once the process of fertilization results in the constitution of a zygote through the union of the human egg and sperm.

In giving her moral teachings, which I personally accept, the Church generally refers to the zygote or the product of fertilization as a human being, a human subject with rights and even a human person but without intending to commit herself to a statement of a philosophical character. In other words, the Church has gone as far as she possibly could without expressly declaring that the zygote is a human individual in the philosophical sense of a human being or human person, personally identical with the fetus, future infant, child and adult. Consequently though different stages of development of the human individual are recognized, the Church places them all on the one ethical level:

> The terms 'zygote', 'pre-embryo', 'embryo' and 'foetus' can indicate in the vocabulary of biology successive stages of the development of a living human being. This Instruction makes free use of these terms, attributing to them an identical ethical relevance, in order to designate the fruit (whether capable of autonomous life or not) of a human generation, from the first moment of its existence until birth.[108]

After quoting parts of paragraphs 12 and 13 of the 1974 *Declaration on Procured Abortion*, cited above, the Vatican Instruction continues:

> This teaching remains valid and is further confirmed, if confirmation were needed, by recent findings of human biological science which recognize that in the zygote* resulting from fertilization the biological identity of a new human individual is already constituted.
>
> Certainly no experimental datum can be in itself sufficient to bring us to the recognition of a spiritual soul; nevertheless, the conclusions of science regarding the human embryo provide valuable indications for discerning by the use of reason a personal presence from this first appearance of a human life: how could a living human creature not be a human person? The Magisterium has expressly not committed its authority to this affirmation of a philosophical nature, but it constantly reaffirms the moral condemnation of any kind of procured abortion. This teaching has not been changed and is unchangeable.
>
> Thus the fruit of human generation, from the first moment of its existence, that is from when the formation of the zygote begins, demands the absolute respect that is morally due to man in his bodily and spiritual totality. The human creature is to be respected and treated as a person from the moment of conception; and therefore from that same moment his rights as a person should be recognized, among which in the first place is the inviolable right of every innocent human creature to life.
>
> *The zygote is the cell that arises from the fusion of two gametes.[109]

Further on we find the following:

> Human embryos obtained *in vitro* are to be considered human creatures and subjects with rights: their dignity and right to life must be respected from the first moment of their existence.[110]

As mentioned above, the Congregation for the Doctrine of the Faith is aware of the philosophical discussions in course concerning the beginning of the human person. Certain distinctions have to be tested philosophically for their validity and relevance in regard to the origin of the human person. The Church knows more discussions are needed to clarify the notions of biological or genetic human individuality, ontological individuality and the requirements of a continuing ontological identity in relation to a human person from his or her outset. The Church is not yet prepared to give definitive teaching of a philosophical nature on precisely when a human person begins. In the meantime she assumes the human person begins at fertilization and relies on philosophers, in dialogue with modern science, to critically investigate these matters with a high sense of moral responsibility in order to suggest a convincing answer to this sensitive question of when the human person begins. The onus is on authors, like myself, to prove that the commonly accepted assumptions of the broader community and of the Church lack the necessary biological and philosophical support.

12   Conclusion

It is my conviction that whoever wishes to tackle the question of the origin of the individual human being cannot dispense with the study of the history of the problem over the last two and a half thousand years. The insights to be gained are invaluable. They highlight the need to continue the search for a solution within the framework of sound philosophical principles and in the light of all the evidence available from early human embryology. This is all the more necessary when we see that the teachings of the Bible and the Church give practical guidance and motivation for acting morally in relation to life issues rather than answer explicitly in philosophical terms the question of when a human individual begins.

3

Criteria for being a human individual

1   Ordinary knowledge of human individuals

Our knowledge of things in the world is at first global and generic before progressing to become more specific. Most of our ordinary knowledge is expressed by predicating something of an object. This is usually called the logical subject. Thus when I say 'The cat is black', I know something about 'the cat' that is the logical subject of the statement. The logical subject refers to something that exists in the world of experience of the speaker. This ability to refer to something as really given in our world is the simplest form of knowledge that we have, e.g. 'The cat ....' Admittedly, this sort of knowledge does not tell us very much unless we say something else, i.e. predicate something about it thereby expanding our knowledge of it. If we can only refer to something and are unable to know anything more about it, we can say that it is there or here. For example, 'There's a cat' or 'A cat is here' or, at least, 'Something is here'.

The knowledge involved in our ability to refer to an object is indeed imperfect, but it is knowledge of a sort that serves as a starting point for acquiring more knowledge about it. Our ability to refer to things is the launching pad for all our further intellectual explorations. Crucial to the building up of knowledge is our ability to differentiate between the various objects encountered in our experience. This enables them to become the logical subjects of our thoughts without running the risk of constant confusion. In ordinary discourse we say something about what we refer to or talk about. In other words, we predicate about the logical subjects of our sentences. In the example given above we say that the cat is black, 'is black' being predicated of 'the cat' that is referred to. In this way, not only do we manage to predicate, we can even progress far enough to give accurate descriptions of what we refer to, if not definitions themselves.

People all over the world, young and old, are able to refer successfully to human individuals. In most cases something true can also be predicated of them even if it is not necessarily something profound. Humans can easily be distinguished from horses, dogs and other animals. This does not imply that all those who can make an identifying reference to a human person would be able to give an accurate description of one, much less a definition. Our descriptions of human individuals improve with time. Our ability to predicate essential characteristics of human individuals grows with our own self-understanding, our experience of inter-personal relationships, our education and our cultural standards. Familiarity with some basic philosophical concepts would clearly enhance our ability to grasp the meaning of a human individual in greater depth and breadth. This would certainly be required if we were to speak of the predicament of human existence.

This does not mean that the ordinary person who has not studied philosophy does not understand what a human person is. We should not confuse the basic and original knowledge of human individuals displayed in our successful predications about them as logical subjects, with a comprehensive account of what it means to be a human person in philosophical terms. The average citizen, no less than the philosopher, can recognize and identify a live human individual, a human person. Any acceptable philosophical definition of a human person must accord with the common-sense understanding of ordinary people. There is no club of people with particular characteristics that can make an exclusive claim to be human individuals or to recognize human individuals. The illiterate and the erudite are all equally human and all are aware of this fact.

Our ordinary concept of human person is based on our understanding of a human being, a human individual. None of us has ever met a person that was not an individual human being. We cannot explain what a person is without reference to our knowledge of human beings gained through experience. It is only by analogy that we extend this notion to *divine persons* or persons by legal fiction, e.g. colleges, corporations, political parties, etc. Jenny Teichman makes her point clearly:

> The reasons for calling some entity a person always refer back to behaviour or (as Wittgenstein might say) to the natural history of human beings. Conversely, it would be ludicrous to be asked to give one's reasons for supposing that human beings are persons. If human beings are not persons, then, one is inclined to say, there can be no such things as persons at all.... Immature, defective,

sick and dying human beings all count as persons not only in Law, but in the way we talk. Anyone who wishes to deny personhood to what in fact are human beings (for instance to foreigners, or to people in coma) invariably denies humanity as well.[1]

We usually refer to a living member of our species in common conversation as *Homo sapiens* or as a *human individual* or a *human being*. Ordinary people and common linguistic usage also employ the term *person*, understood as a natural person. The *Oxford Dictionary* agrees where it gives the meaning of the term *person* as 'individual human being'. There is no doubt in my mind that all three expressions may refer equally to a member of our human species. For the purposes of defining legal rights and protection, the natural meaning of the term *person* may be restricted in law to refer to a human individual that is alive after birth. This does not mean that there is no living human individual prior to birth. For the purposes of this book, we may disregard the legal interpretation of the term *person* since we are primarily concerned with when a human individual begins, not legal definitions. Though some philosophers further restrict the meaning of the term natural *person* and/or human being, as we shall see, I shall use all three ways of referring to the members of our biological species *Homo sapiens* as interchangeable and with the same meaning – human individual, human being and person.

Philosophical reflection can be of great assistance in clarifying our ordinary concept of the human individual without in any way being untrue to it. This is to be our next task in relation to our understanding of the adult human individual before attempting to determine when the human individual begins. An approach is said to be *subjective* if it proceeds from the perspective of the person or subject concerned. Otherwise it is said to be *objective*. In the case of research into drugs, a subjective approach would describe them in terms of how it feels to experience them, whereas an objective method would describe their chemical constitution as well as their biological and psychological effects. Both approaches may be employed in the case of humans. The distinction between both approaches is valid even if it is made in terms of human thinking.

First we shall try to grasp the meaning of a human being from within the perspective of the self-conscious human individual. This is variously called the experiential, personalist or even subject-centred approach to analysing the meaning of personhood. This will be followed by considerations of a more metaphysical kind, that try to explain how a human individual must be objectively constituted to account for the unique self-conscious experience enjoyed by persons. Finally, an attempt will be made to give a definition of a human person that is applicable from the very beginning of the human individual.

2   Personalist understanding of the human individual

From within ourselves we understand that we are unique, quite distinct from other persons and things. Though each one of us is a self, we also experience ourselves as members of a community of others like ourselves. Even if one were to exist alone on an island, one could conceive that others might exist like oneself with whom one could relate. In other words, we soon learn that we *are* social by nature (even if we occasionally fail to act socially). We are aware of the basic difference in meaning between *being* and *having*. We *have* things that are not part of ourselves, but we *are* ourselves. Yet we still say that we *have* a body and at the same time are *a body* in the sense that we *are* corporeal beings. The self can both identify with the body and withdraw somewhat from the body by way of *having* it. The self or personal *ego* cannot be known directly for the simple reaon that it only becomes aware of itself, through its conscious activities. These conscious acts reveal the self as the subject of both bodily and non-bodily activities. The same self may be conscious of both a predominantly bodily activity like walking and a rather non-bodily or mental activity like thinking. The same human individual who is walking may also be thinking. Our basic awareness is of the self as one whole complex being that is the subject and originating source of both corporeal and non-corporeal activities alike.

Our thinking acts may include making important judgments of fact or even making judgments of conscience that we experience as morally binding on ourselves. Such acts are experienced as closer to the very core of our being and personhood than acts like walking or scratching. We also experience acts that we regard as free and for which we hold ourselves morally responsible. Acts of love of our neighbour that cost us some sacrifice would rank high amongst our free acts that likewise come close to the core of ourselves as individual human beings. It is in trying to be true to ourselves in all our acts that we seek happiness and self-fulfillment. We recognize that our dignity and value reside in ourselves in as much as we are subjects capable of desiring and enjoying genuine lasting happiness. We intuitively know that we are worth more than animals and that we may not be reduced to the status of mere objects or means for others' purposes. The resentment and offence we experience when others abuse us loudly proclaims our sense of the absolute and inviolable character of the dignity and value of the whole of our being as an end in itself. I believe there can be little dispute with this account of how we perceive ourselves as persons in the subjective mode of thinking. This is what appears in our consciousness. We often use the term *personality* to refer to how we perceive human individuals expressing themselves as persons. Its meaning is akin to the subjective perspective of human personhood, including individual characteristics, moral character, psychological traits, cultural outlook, social awareness.

John Locke (d.1704) proposes a similar analysis, not for man, but for person. Man's identity would be determined more by biological criteria, whereas for him a person is one who can engage personal faculties:

> We must consider what *person* stands for: – which I think is a thinking intelligent being, that has reason and reflection, and can consider itself as itself, the same thinking thing, in different times and places; which it does only by that consciousness which is inseparable from thinking, and, as it seems to me, essential to it: it being impossible for anyone to perceive without *perceiving* that he does perceive. When we see, hear, smell, taste, feel, meditate, or will anything, we know that we do so... *Person*, as I take it, is the name for this self. Wherever a man finds what he calls himself, there, I think, another may say is the same person. It is a forensic term, appropriating actions and their merit; and so belongs only to intelligent agents, capable of a law, and happiness, and misery.[2]

We find Locke here practically defining a person as a human individual that is a morally or legally responsible agent. We ourselves and the courts have to use discretion to determine whether a particular human individual is, or was, capable of performing morally and/or legally responsible actions.

Peter Strawson is close to Locke, but gives more importance to the body conceived as a subject of conscious states and experiences that can be predicated both of the self and of others on logically adequate criteria. His concept of a person is as follows:

> What I mean by the concept of a person is the concept of a type of entity such that *both* predicates ascribing states of consciousness *and* predicates ascribing corporeal characteristics, a physical situation etc. are equally applicable to a single individual of that single type ... a necessary condition of states of consciousness

being ascribed at all is that they should be ascribed to the *very
same things* as corporeal characteristics, a certain physical
situation etc.[3]

Peter Singer speaks of person as 'a rational self-conscious being',[4] while
Michael Tooley holds a similar view requiring a person to be a 'subject of
non-momentary interests'.[5] Singer subsequently expressed his views more
fully on his concept of person, proposing a more restricted concept of a
human being as:

> ...a being possessing, at least at a minimal level, the capacities
> distinctive of our species, which include consciousness, the ability
> to be aware of one's surroundings, the ability to relate to others,
> perhaps even rationality and self-consciousness.[6]

Michael Lockwood says much the same thing:

> A person is a being that is conscious, in the sense of having the
> capacity for conscious thought and experiences, but not only that:
> it must have the capacity for reflective consciousness and self-
> consciousness. It must have, or at any rate have the ability to
> acquire, a concept of itself, as a being with a past and a future.
> Mere sentience is not enough to qualify as being a person.[7]

John Harris likewise does not go beyond what is given immediately in
experience for his definition:

> A person will thus be any individual capable of valuing its own
> life. Such a being will, at the very least, be able to conceive of itself
> as an independent centre of consciousness, existing over time with
> a future that it is capable of envisaging and wishing to
> experience.[8]

Baroness Warnock in reviewing John Harris' concept of person, based
on the capacity to value one's own life, also discusses a person as a bearer
of rights. In other words, a person is one that ought to be respected. If a
person is taken in this sense, one then asks when ought one begin to respect
a human individual, implying there is a time in its development when an
individual might not be worthy of absolute respect. She does not believe it
is at all helpful to ask when does a new life begin. This misleads one into
believing there is an observable factual answer to the question of the
beginning of life. The real difficulties involved in finding a satisfactory
answer suggest 'the question of what counts as a new life [is] unanswerable
in principle'.[9]

We are left with the question when does human life begin to morally matter or, simply, when does a person begin? Again, difficulties arise in determining the appropriate moral principles and criteria for deciding when respect should be shown to the developing human individual, i.e. when does a person begin. Ordinary usage, as well as the legal employment, of the term *person* compound the problem and make one believe there is an exact answer that could be discovered by research for the beginning of personhood. Baroness Warnock finds it is practically impossible to decide what is to count as a person in general on the criteria of rationality and self-value. Could one really say a fetus values itself or its life? She concludes it would be better to side-step the concept of person and go straight to the real point at issue and ask how ought a human individual or embryo be treated and on what agreed moral principles should such treatment be based.[10]

Baroness Warnock recently summarized her position on this point quite clearly, showing also the thinking behind the stand adopted in the Warnock Report quoted above (see p. 4):

> For the question about *moral significance*, the question, that is, *when do embryos morally matter*, is quite obviously one that must be answered by judgment and decision, according to a particular moral standpoint. It is not a question of fact but a question of value. How much *should* we value a human life in its very early stages? But to translate this into a question about whether or not in the early stages an embryo *is a person* looks like translating this question into a question of fact. It looks as if by inspecting the embryo and finding out what features it has, we could discover a non-controversial answer. That personhood, its possession or non-possession, is as much a question of value as is the question when human life begins to matter, is hard for people to grasp. And yet it is manifestly the case....
>
> I believe that the only way out of the difficulty is the short one: to bypass the concept of the person altogether. After all, the notion was introduced only on the grounds that persons are the bearers of rights. Since there seems no separately satisfactory way of distinguishing a person from a non-person, apart from their supposedly having rights, it seems better to take the direct route forward and ask whether or not human embryos have rights.[11]

It is taken for granted by all these authors that the human person is also a member of the species *Homo sapiens*. They agree, however, that being biologically human does not suffice to count as a human person. The active capacity for exercising some minimally self-conscious rational acts must have already been acquired by the developing human individual. It is necessary to bear in mind the meaning of the term 'person' for these modern philosophers in order to avoid serious misunderstandings. Their concept of person does not accord with the common understanding of person employed in ordinary linguistic usage. It is confusing to use it with this meaning as opposed to 'human being' or 'human individual'.

3   Metaphysical understanding of the human individual

A personalist account needs to be complemented to give a complete philosophical exposition of the human person. Some metaphysical explanation in the objective mode of thinking is essential. A metaphysical understanding of the human individual must start with the acceptance of all the basic facts of our experience outlined above. The fundamental unity of the self as the single subject of all our experiences, whether they be corporeal or not, is of paramount importance. This non-dualistic constitution of the human individual needs stressing. In addition to stating this psychosomatic unity of mind and body, an explanation is needed to show how this is possible in terms of philosophical principles. It is not enough to point to the unity in our concept of person as Strawson does. It is necessary to seek a theory that will explain how one individual being can really be the subject of both corporeal and conscious states.

There can be no denying some sort of dualism in the human individual. At the same time this dualism does not detract from the real unity of each human being that primarily exists as the subject of both kinds of activities, namely, physical and conscious. The term *ontological individual* is used by philosophers to refer to a single thing that exists in itself and not merely as a real part or principle of a greater whole. It is an independent being that exists in its own right. An ontological individual may also be referred to as a material subject of existence, a concrete reality, as one material thing among others, or more simply as a concrete entity. Obviously, one individual cannot be another.

Granted the person is a single entity, its unity can only be explained in terms of distinct principles that are not themselves separate things, but real co-principles of a human individual that actually exists. There are degrees of real existence. Being real does not imply separate individual existence. Any sort of dualism is ruled out that would mean a union of two distinct things or entities instead of a single being. Principles of being are real because they share in the reality of an existing individual. The separation of body and soul espoused by Plato and Descartes does not ring true to the multi-faceted unity experienced by ourselves as personal subjects. No explanation of the two dimensions of the human person is satisfactory that *de facto* would deny the obvious unity attested to by our ordinary experience. The real dual polarity of body and soul must not be taken as though it was inconsistent with the basic oneness of a human being. A multiplicity of qualities is quite compatible with the ontological unity of the human person. The unity of any existent individual must take precedence over any real distinctions that might be introduced by a theory to explain the various characteristics and activities of the one and the same individual.

One satisfactory way to explain the unity of the human individual is the Aristotelian hylomorphic theory of *matter* and *form* where the soul is the *form* of the body. Matter and soul are principles of being, not things themselves that exist separately prior to the coming into existence of the human individual. In fact, the human individual exists by virtue of the matter and soul related to each other as potency to actuality within the unity of a single being or entity. This hylomorphic account of the constitution of the human individual adequately explains the dual polarity of the human person as the subject of activities and predicates that are predominately corporeal or non-corporeal. The soul is one with the body, forming, determining, actuating and organizing the matter to be a human body, including all its tissues, organs, limbs and sexuality. The body is the subject of all our conscious activities and shares in the unique sense of dignity and value of the human being in every way. This represents a metaphysical explanation of the human nature of each person, where soul and matter constitute a single ontological individual.

The hylomorphic theory explains how it is possible for death to occur when a living animal changes into a corpse. The very concept of change implies that something common remains the same and something different or new appears. Death occurs when a specific form is no longer able to actuate the matter to be a living animal and yields to a new form(s) that arises from the potency of the same matter to make a corpse.[12] A human being also dies when the soul is no longer able to actuate his/her matter. The matter changes from one type of being to another because it is able to do so, given the right conditions. If matter was unable to become something different, there could be no change of being from one type to another. There would be no death at all. Matter of its nature is substantially mutable. The hylomorphic theory of matter and form provides an explanation for the possibility of intrinsic change in all types of material things, from death in the organic world (including humans) to similar substantial changes in the inorganic world (e.g. water becoming hydrogen and oxygen).

The theory of matter and form also explains how it is possible to have multiple instances of individuals of the same type of material being or substance. While it is true that there are many human individuals, it is also true that they are identical in species or type of being. The problem is the same for many instances of crystals, hydrogen atoms or molecules of water. We need to explain the possibility both of the multiplicity of individuals as well as of the unity of the same type of being. They obviously differ in their matter even if we are dealing with identical individuals that are actuated by the same type of form, e.g. identical human twins or molecules of water. One twin is really distinct from the other: the matter of one is not that of the other. It is quantified matter that accounts for the possibility of the same type of individual being produced again and again by the same type of form. Science itself presupposes that distinct individuals or instances of the same type of substance have the same nature all over the world. Hydrogen and oxygen interact and unite to form water in Australia as well as in England. Human individuals in all five continents have the same human nature notwithstanding differences in race, size, age, colour or other characteristics. The species–individual structure of things argues in favour of the hylomorphic theory of matter and form in as much as matter has the potential to be actuated by the same form many times over to give origin to many distinct quantified individuals with the same type of nature.[13]

The potentiality of matter explains the fundamental mutability of material beings. This enables them to change from one type to another, given the right conditions and the activation of the appropriate causes. The same potentiality of matter enables many individuals of the same type of species to exist in distinct masses of quantified matter. The hylomorphic theory does not remove the mystery of the unity of matter and soul in humans. There will always be mysteries when we try to explain the constitution of any individual being in philosophical terms. I believe the Aristotelian hylomorphic theory is a step in the right direction to explain the fundamental psychosomatic unity of soul and matter within the ontological unity of the human individual.

Many philosophers believe the human person can be satisfactorily explained in purely empirical terms. According to this view, the human individual is just a living body that has the capacity to engage in rational self-conscious acts. Human beings can be adequately explained in terms of the properties of matter and material energy in much the same way that we explain the constitution and behaviour of animals. It follows that after death occurs a human being completely ceases to exist. Materialistic philosophers could equally use the hylomorphic theory to account for death in a human being as in an animal since the soul would be no more than a material form. In this case once a person died his/her form would be reduced to the potency of matter and consequently cease to exist as in any other instance of substantial change.

Many other philosophers, myself included, do not believe the constitution and activities of the human person can be adequately explained in terms of matter and material energy alone. Whereas an animal can only *see* green grass, a person can *see* and *assert that* the grass *is* green. This means that we can know that it is true to say that the grass is green. When we assert some truth, we imply that we know some particular aspect of reality. This happens whenever we predicate something of a logical subject in realistic discourse, namely when the subject really exists. The knowledge of truth expressed in simple predications reveals a typically human capacity of reflective self-awareness. It is this intellectual power that enables us to be aware of ourselves as persons and moral agents, acting with, or without, a sense of dignity, in all our reflective self-conscious acts. This applies not only to acts of knowledge but also to free non-cognitive human acts that express love, hatred, joy, sorrow, sympathy, anger or greed. A sense of moral responsibility for our acts presupposes this capacity of rational self-consciousness.

Human knowledge goes far beyond the capacity of an animal's perception that is restricted to objects, associations and relationships that fall within its perceptual field or its possible imaginary projections. We have an unrestricted notion of reality that we employ to make true statements both in empirical and non-empirical discourse (e.g. about God). Our rational self-consciousness and typically human knowledge distinguish us from animals. The total self-presence implied in such acts cannot be explained in terms of quantified matter alone nor in space–time categories. This is why a non-material life-principle or soul is required in a human being to function as an ordinary form to account for the psychosomatic unity of the one subject of all human activities. It is no surprise to find the human individual referred to as 'an incarnated spirit', 'an embodied soul' or 'an animated body'.

4   The same human individual as an adult or infant person

We should now try to attempt a provisional definition of a human being that includes a reference to both the metaphysical and the personalist dimensions discussed above. It could run as follows: a human individual is a member of our species *Homo sapiens*, who on account of a unique psychosomatic constitution, is capable of experiencing self-conscious, rational and free acts in addition to performing nutritive and physiological functions and other bodily activities. This definition would satisfy most of us most of the time for most purposes in life. When we talk about persons we usually refer to people who are capable of experiencing self-conscious rational acts. Yet nobody would dream of excluding somebody who was asleep or unconscious from the class of human individuals. We spontaneously recognize that being an individual with the ability to exercise typically human rational acts suffices to constitute a person, not necessarily the actual exercising of such acts. Consequently, we need to broaden our definition of the human individual accordingly.

We have seen above how some philosophers think that personhood merely consists in human self-conscious and rational activities or, at least, in an acquired ability to exercise them. This is an important point to clarify for all, especially infants. The following lines of Helga Kuhse and Peter Singer indicate that this is no mere hypothetical academic discussion:

> We must recall, however, that when we kill a new-born infant there is no *person* whose life has begun. When I think of myself as the person I now am, I realize that I did not come into existence until sometime after my birth. At birth I had no sense of the future, and no experiences which I can now remember as 'mine'. It is the beginning of the life of the person, rather than of the physical organism, that is crucial so far as the right to life is concerned.[14]

If we reflect a little, we realize that our pleasant and painful experiences, in short all our self-conscious acts, do not exist in themselves. They only exist as experiences and activities of the human individual that is their subject. They express the being of the human individual. Self-consciousness brings this home to us very vividly. It makes us aware of ourselves as human subjects of experiences and activities. We cannot drive a wedge between conscious experiences and the subject who has them. Personhood or personal individuality continues when rational activities cease during sleep because it is one with the human individual that is the subject of all its self-conscious and rational activities. This allows us to re-identify ourselves as the same persons from day to day. The human individual continues to exist and endure with a nature that enables it to express itself in self-conscious and rational acts. In fact, we can truly say that personhood consists in the natural capacity of a human individual to express itself through various functions and activities, especially self-conscious rational and free acts.

The sound judgment of people the world over recognizes that new-born babies are human persons, even though they have not yet developed to the stage of having acquired the ability to exercise self-conscious rational acts. This acknowledgement is universally encoded in civil and criminal law. The basis for this recognition of the personal status of the infant is surely to be found in the fact that it is the same individual being that gradually grows and develops into the adult human individual. Nobody doubts the personal and moral status of the human adult. In the case of an infant we are dealing with an identity in being, i.e. a continuing ontological identity from birth onwards, notwithstanding subsequent development of limbs, organs and the brain to the age of reason and beyond. Each one of us recognizes that we are the *same being* today that was born many years ago. A birth certificate states something about oneself, not another from whom one emerged through a developmental process.

This is an extremely important judgment by mankind about a human person's ontological identity beginning at least at birth and continuing unchanged as growth and development take place over the years. No philosophical definition of a person can discount this fact of ordinary human experience. The courts themselves take this for granted in cases of homicide, inheritance and suing for damages suffered in infancy. *It is understood that the infant has an inherent natural active capacity to develop to the stage of being able to exercise self-conscious and rational acts while retaining the same ontological identity as a human individual.* We can simply and truly sum things up by saying that *a person is a living individual with a truly human nature, i.e. a human individual, a human being. An infant is a person already because its nature enables it to develop to the age of reason without loss of ontological identity.*

In the case of the new-born baby, we know that we are in the presence of an actual human individual endowed with the potential to develop, in due time, all its natural abilities, given the right conditions of nourishment, care and environment. The growth and development of an infant is the growth and development of a human being to maturity, not growth and development into a human being. The developing infant gradually realizes its natural potential to express more fully what it already is. It does not grow into something else. The development of one individual being is not development into another kind of individual being. The same ontological reality, the same identical being continues in existence throughout growth. We do not have the formation of a different ontological individual.

If *Michael* is a new-born male infant, it is the same *Michael* that grows to become a child, acquires the age of reason and the ability to predicate, reaches puberty and a marriageable age, marries and eventually becomes a father. We can say that *Michael* remains the same ontological individual throughout all these developmental stages. The new-born infant *Michael* is a person with potential to grow, not simply a potential person. This philosophical interpretation of the human individual's ontological identity corresponds with the common-sense view of the human person continuing from birth to death with the same identity. It is not simply a matter of wishing this to be so: we recognize this is the case. It is quite different in the case of grape juice. It is not wine, but only potentially wine. In the same way everybody admits the human sperm and egg are not a human being, but they jointly have the potential to become a human being, given fertilization, time, development and the right conditions.

One either is or is not a human being. There can be no place for a 'no man's land' in this case. We are all equally human beings once we are constituted as living individuals with a human nature. We do vary in our level of intelligence – high, average or low. This does not change the fact that we are all equally human persons. The fact that the intelligence of a chimpanzee or dolphin may be greater than that of a new born infant does not make any animal qualify for personal status. Our personhood has its foundation in the living individual's human nature, including its bio- logical dimensions. No animal has a human nature nor is any endowed with a human being's specific natural capacities. Personhood does not exist apart from a living individual's human nature. We cannot divorce personhood from a human nature. In this regard I cannot agree with those philosophers who suggest dolphins and chimpanzees are non-human persons.[15] It is not helpful to disregard what the ordinary reasonable man or woman understands by the term *person* by conferring personal status on animals outside the context of fairy tales or cartoons.

The timing of the beginning of the human individual actually coincides with ensoulment itself. The soul must not be thought of as something apart from the human individual because it is the form of the human body. Consequently the soul does not have a separate beginning from that of the living individual with a human nature. When an infant reaches the age of reason and becomes capable of performing the self-reflective conscious and free acts of a moral agent there is no question of a new individual coming into existence. The infant is the same living individual as the child, with the same ontological identity. The life-principle of the new-born infant is the same as that of the growing child and the adult with the full use of the power of reason. There is no evidence to believe a *new* life-principle or a *new* individual begins at the age of reason. On the contrary, empirical evidence interpreted in the light of sound philosophical principles argues quite convincingly in favour of the infant growing into the child and the adult without loss of ontological individuality. There are only new rational self-conscious expressions of the same human individual.

It must be remembered that the soul is a non-material or spiritual life-principle that is required to explain the non-quantitative aspects of rational self-conscious acts of knowledge and free choice. Purely empirical methods of investigation cannot be used to observe directly the presence of the soul as such, nor the beginning of its presence. Philosophical reasoning is required to establish the necessity of a soul to explain the rational and free acts of human individuals. It is pointless to ask when ensoulment occurs unless it is taken to also ask when a new human individual begins, endowed by the Creator with a soul. We can justifiably conclude that the soul that animates the adult human individual animates the infant right from the beginning of its existence as a living ontological individual with a human nature. As we shall soon see, this applies not only to the new-born infant but also to the fetus prior to birth.

The absence of rational activity in the human adult during sleep and comatose states does not prove the absence of a spiritual soul. It simply means a sleeping or comatose person lacks, for the time being, the requisite favourable organic physiological and neurological conditions required for the expression of human acts that are self-conscious, rational, free and moral. In the case of the new-born infant, the soul would indeed be present, but rational self-conscious acts could not be performed prior to the development and presence of those same requisite favourable organic physiological and neurological conditions. The newly born baby already has the capacity to acquire the ability to perform rational acts.

5   The human individual prior to birth

There can be little doubt that the fetus in the mother's womb is a human individual prior to birth once it is admitted that the new-born infant is a human being. The child that is born is the same developing human individual that was in the mother's womb. Birth alone cannot confer natural personhood or human individuality. This is confirmed by premature deliveries of babies who are as truly human and almost as viable as those whose gestation goes to full term. Being viable inside or outside the mother's womb makes a difference to the kind of dependence required for survival, not a difference to being a human individual or not. Viability outside the womb cannot be advanced as a genuine intrinsic criterion for being a human individual. The fetus that is only viable within the womb is already a distinct human individual, even if it depends on the mother to continue living. In any case, viability outside the womb is too arbitrary. A low birth-weight baby born in a hospital equipped with a neo-natal intensive care unit would most likely survive, whereas the same baby born elsewhere without the same expert care and sophisticated facilities would most likely die. All the evidence and reason itself support the human fetus prior to birth being a true ontological human individual and consequently a human person in fact if not in law.

We have already seen Lockwood's concept of person. His concept of 'human being' comes between that of person and 'human organism' taken simply in the biological sense of a complete living organism of the species *Homo sapiens*.[16] For Lockwood the term human being stands for:

> ...whatever it is that you and I are essentially, what we can neither become nor cease to be, without ceasing to exist.[17]

He means that a human being may become a person and still remain a human being. A non-personal human being may develop into a person, a personal human being. There is continuity of identity between a human being and a person, whereas there is no such continuity of identity between the biological living organism of the human species and the human being and the human person. In Lockwood's view a week-old human embryo is neither a human being nor a person.[18]

A human being according to Lockwood, cannot begin before the appropriate brain structures are developed that are capable of sustaining awareness. Their continuity in time constitutes the continuing identity of the human being by providing its continuous physical underpinning.[19] He explains his position as follows:

> Just as I shall live only as long as the relevant part of my brain remains essentially intact, so I came into existence only when the appropriate part or parts of my brain came into existence, or more precisely, reached the appropriate stage of development to sustain my identity as a human being, with the capacity for consciousness. When I came into existence is a matter of how far

back the relevant neurophysiological continuity can be traced. Presumably, then, my life began somewhere between conception and birth.[20]

No doubt a functioning brain is a pre-requisite for the exercise of self-conscious, rational and free acts. States of sleep, coma and damage to the cerebral hemispheres bear this out. There can be no immediate potential for rational activity unless one is awake with a functioning brain. This does not mean, however, there could be no human individual prior to the presence of a functioning brain. Once there is a biologically human organism that, without loss of ontological identity, has the potential to develop all that is necessary for eventually exercising typically human self-conscious rational acts, there is a true human individual.

Lockwood is right in suggesting we need something by way of a subject to support our conscious states. The human individual is the subject of our existence, our rational nature and of all our powers, parts and activities. The brain is not the subject of our conscious states. The brain is not conscious, but the human individual is conscious, thanks to a functioning brain. The human individual is also the subject of the functioning brain's activities. This is what Aristotle would call an individual substance, that which primarily exists and in which all attributes of the relevant individual substance, or entity, subsist and inhere. It is a matter of thinking about the fundamental bearer or subject of existence. This is what really counts. In our case, it is the person, the human being, the human individual. This way of viewing things also corresponds to ordinary common-sense realism. It is such a simple insight that we seldom talk about it; we just take it for granted. On the other hand Lockwood's concept of the human being really lacks convincing evidence. A human organism understood as an ontological individual with a continuing identity would suffice to count as a human being and to support personal and rational acts from the onset of the age of reason.

There can be no comparison between the situation of a human adult dying from irreversible cessation of all brain activity and that of an embryonic human individual whose inherent active potential to develop a functioning brain remains intact. In the latter case the presence of the same developing human individual is becoming more apparent, while in the former it is fading away as general organic disintegration yields a lifeless corpse. Once living matter forms an ontological individual and begins to actualize its natural potential for human development with the same ontological identity, that individual already has a human nature. It would already be a human being with potential, not a potential human being.

Stages and degrees of development and growth are not prejudicial to the continuing presence of the same human individual provided an ontological human individual existed in the first place. It must at least be able to begin to realize its natural human potential. It must have the natural capacity, given a suitable environment, nourishment and other favourable conditions, to begin to develop and grow towards the adult stage of life and to acquire the ability to exercise the typically human activities of self-conscious, rational, free and moral acts. All the activities of a human individual express his/her condition and stage of development. This is particularly true of the fetus. The same applies to a deformed fetus. It would still be a human individual even if its human nature was not perfect nor its functions quite normal. Once an individual with a true human nature begins to exist and develop, it continues to be a human individual while it is alive, even if severe congenital malformations occur subsequently during development. Nobody questions the humanity of a Down's syndrome fetus or child. A fetus or child with severe open *spina bifida* is nonetheless a human being. The same should be said of the live anencephalic fetus or infant with only brain stem functions: it is a human individual even if it lacks a complete brain and usually survives birth by only a few hours or a day.

Quite different is the case of the placental abnormality known as the hydatidiform mole, composed of grape-like clusters of swollen chorionic villi. It was known in antiquity. It is the product of an abnormal fertilization where live placental tissue is formed without any embryo at all. All 46 chromosomes are derived from the father, with no genetic contribution coming from the mother. This usually happens as a result of a single haploid sperm fertilizing an egg where the pronucleus is either absent or non-functional. After entry, the chromosomes of the sperm double up, giving rise to the diploid number of 46 chromosomes in a mole that is homozygous for all its paternal genes.[21] Though the mole is alive and of human origin, it is definitely not a human individual or human being. Unlike the anencephalic fetus it lacks a true human nature from the start and has no natural potential to begin human development (see Fig. 3.1).

A *teratoma* is a new abnormal and uncontrolled growth of cells and tissue. This is another clear instance of cells developing abnormally that result from the product of fertilization, but which could not be considered to be a true human individual with a human nature. It has no potential to develop into an entire fetus or infant. It represents a serious error in the

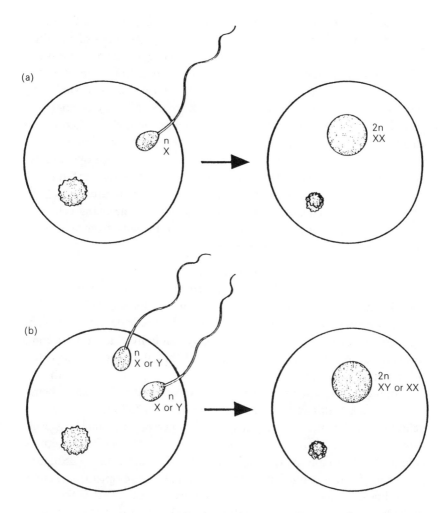

Fig. 3.1. Diagram to illustrate the origin of hydatidiform moles. (*a*) A single haploid spermatozoon fertilizes an oocyte with a defective pronucleus which takes no part in the fertilization process. The chromosomes of the spermatozoon double up, to give a diploid zygote that is therefore homozygous for all paternal genes. The fact that no YY moles are found suggests that at least one X chromosome is essential for life, even in a molar trophoblast. (*b*) Two haploid spermatozoa, either X- and Y-bearing or both X-bearing, fertilize an oocyte with a defective nucleus which takes no part in the fertilization process. The two male pronuclei subsequently fuse to give a heterozygous diploid zygote. This mode of origin accounts for some if not all the XY moles (4 per cent of all moles), and probably also for a small proportion of the XX moles. (Reproduced with permission from *Embryonic and Fetal Development, Reproduction in mammals* Bk 2, C. R. Austin and R. V. Short, Cambridge University Press, 1982.)

reproductive and developmental process. It may occur in the ovary or the testis. At times a teratoma develops from pluripotent cells of primitive streak origin. In this case the living teratoma may contain various types of tissues due to chaotic cell development. It may contain remnants of several organs forming an amalgam of disorganized fetal parts, e.g. tissue, bone, hair, teeth, etc.[22] Clearly, such a disorganized mass of living cells could not itself be the subject of an individual's human nature whether it was attached to a living fetal human individual or existed apart from a fetus. An attached teratoma would be more akin to a cancerous tumour invading the human individual than a live part of it. Clearly, the fetus with the teratoma would be a human individual, but not the teratoma itself. Its importance for our purpose is to note that not all the living cells that develop from the conceptus, the early embryo or the fetus form an integral part of a developing human individual.

6   The traditional concept of person

The concept of the human person that emerges from these considerations of the development of the human individual both before and after birth is quite similar to the traditional classic definition given by the medieval philosopher Boethius, namely, 'an individual substance in a rational nature'. It was taken for granted that the concrete individual substance would be alive and consequently capable of growth and development. The rational nature referred to was that of the human being. Aquinas makes this clear when he comments as follows on Boethius' definition: 'It belongs to every man to be a person in as much as every subject in a human nature is a person.'[23] He further clarifies Boethius' definition of person by adding: 'The words "individual substance" appearing in the definition of person signify a complete substance, subsisting in its own right and separately from others.'[24] It is the whole individual substance or entity with a rational nature that is a person. A part of a person is not a person considered independently from the whole person. The arm of a person is not a person taken independently of the whole human individual. Whatever is done by one's arm, moreover, is rightly attributed to the person and not simply to the arm. The whole human person is the subject of the vital functions and the actions freely performed by one's limbs. Our concept of personal responsibility for one's deeds presupposes this.

7   Criteria for the presence of a human individual

We can say the human person is a living individual with a human nature, i.e. a living ontological individual that has within itself the active capacity to maintain, or at least to begin, the process of the human life-cycle without loss of identity. This concept allows the human individual to be the subject of the capacity to develop the ability to exercise, if all goes well, a range of typically human activities, including self-conscious rational, free and moral acts. In other words, *a human person begins as a living individual with the inherent active potential to develop towards human adulthood without ceasing to be the same ontological individual.*

We can remember many events in our lives with accuracy. None of us can remember when we began to be human beings. Quite likely, not even our parents could work that out. Our mothers certainly remember our birthdays, even if we are unable to recall the events. It is not a matter of deciding when *human life* begins. Human life has been transmitted continually for thousands of years. Anthropologists and paleontologists have no precise date for the appearance of human life on our planet. Our task is to find an answer to the question when each one of us began to be a human individual. This is not going to be easy to answer because each person normally begins as an individual at some point during a continuous process of life involving two human individuals – a man and a woman with their gametes.

It may well be beyond us to determine the precise moment when a human individual begins to be. We often are unable to pin-point the precise moment of real death as life gradually ebbs out of a dying person. On the other hand a point does arrive when we know for certain that death has intervened. Death certificates are issued when it is certain death has already occurred. Less certitude exists for the precise moment of death, especially if it has been a slow dying process. This is not to say that there is no precise point when a human individual begins and dies. It is saying that the determination of the precise moment of these events might be beyond us in some instances. Fortunately this does not really matter. For practical purposes it suffices to determine a point in time by which death certainly has occurred before removing organs for transplantation.

We know that the human person is an individual being, or simply an ontological individual. If we are unable to determine precisely when a living individual begins with a human nature, including the soul, we might at least be able to determine a point in the developmental process prior to which it would be impossible or, at least improbable, for an ontological individual with an on-going identity to be formed at all. There cannot be a human person present if the conditions required for the presence of any ontological individual cannot be satisfied. Individuation appears to be the basic criterion. Hence the necessity to clarify the concept of an ontological

individual with reference to inorganic and living ontological individuals
prior to attempting to apply this concept to determining when a human
individual begins. There cannot be a human individual present unless the
criteria for being an individual and a living individual are satisfied. My
criteria are in close agreement with those of John Mahoney, a Jesuit
theologian, who suggests:

> ...that some biological stability in the organism is essential for its
> individuality to be firmly established, and that without this stable
> individuation of the organism one cannot begin to speak of a
> human individual.[25]

We have already seen how Baroness Warnock found it difficult to
disentangle the legal, moral and factual aspects pertaining to the beginning of the human person. She agrees *right treatment* of someone is
relevant to the *who* or *what* in question, suggesting that there are different
degrees of humanness depending on stages of development:

> But I would rather ask whether or not the object of treatment was
> a full human being than whether or not he was a person. 'Human'
> is a biological term, and simply distinguishes humans from other
> animals ... it is clear that there are some members of the species so
> far from full development, so nearly just collections of cells, that
> they do not require full human treatment.[26]

It appears to me she is confusing stages of development in the reproductive process and how the various stages affect our perceptions, feelings
and moral susceptibilities with the blunt fact of whether we are dealing
with a human being or not at all. I say this without prejudice to when a
human individual begins during the reproductive process. Admittedly this
is a question that is difficult to resolve. There must be some answer
philosophers can provide without having recourse to the expedient of an
indiscernible sliding scale of a being that is more or less fully human
instead of a criterion for discerning whether a living ontological individual
is, or is not yet, an individual with a human nature.

8   The concept of an ontological individual

It is now necessary to both clarify and deepen our concept of an
ontological individual to help in our enquiry about the beginning of the
human individual. Earlier I referred to the way our use of language can
cause confusion in relation to the notion of 'conception' itself. Linguistic
usage is moulded to satisfy our ordinary needs of communication as
simply as possible without pretending to express any sophisticated degree

of technical or philosophical expertise in our employment of concepts. The confusion is engendered only if the ordinary use of language is taken to be literally accurate. There is no confusion at all when our use of some logically difficult terms is rendered non-problematical because we are aware that certain linguistic or grammatical features are in-built into their normal employment.

We use many terms in the singular, knowing full well that really they refer to many members of a class or type of being. Think of how we use the following: parliament, crowd, class, herd, hive, forest, litter, bunch or heap. It would be too cumbersome to spell out the actual reference to a multiplicity of members or instances on each occasion. On account of some unifying factor linking all the members together as a whole, we speak in the singular without in any way believing there is no real multiplicity of separate beings involved. Each member of parliament, of the crowd or the class would be an individual, i.e. a single being or entity of the same type or kind as the others included in the meaning of the general term used in the singular.

At other times the unifying factor strikes us more forcefully, especially when we coin a term to refer to a functional unity to serve our purposes of communication. Think of how we speak in the singular of a motor car or a watch. At first sight we might be inclined to think of a car as one thing or entity. We need to reflect before we become aware that the car or watch is really made up of many parts, each of which is a separate thing or entity. The unity in these examples is merely mechanical and functional, serving our needs of transportation or time-keeping. There is no point in speaking of a watch in the plural even though we know it has many really separate parts that are arranged to work together without ceasing to be separate ontological things or individuals existing in their own right by themselves. Once we are alerted to the distinction, we can usually tell the difference between something whose unity is merely artificial, mechanical or functional and something whose natural unity indicates the presence of a single body or an ontological individual. We can readily differentiate between the unity of a bicycle or a train and that of a person, a cat, a tree or a crystal. The latter are true natural ontological individuals whereas the former are not. It is obvious there could not be something with a functional or artificial unity if there were no natural individuals to compose it. There could not be a football team unless it had individual players, nor a sandcastle without individual grains of sand.

The classic definition of an individual given by Aquinas along Aristotelian lines runs as follows: 'An individual is that which is undivided in itself and distinct from others.'[27] The presupposed reference is of course to a material being, not a non-material one. An individual is a natural body that is one subject of existence, notwithstanding the multiplicity of its constituent parts. One whole being actually exists spread out in space on account of its quantified matter. The very nature of extension in an individual requires that one part be not another. What is on the right side cannot be what is on the left side within an individual body. This means that there is a real distinction between one part and another in an individual. But this distinction stops short of being real separation that would result in more than one single individual or entity. Unless matter were capable of being subject to this internal quantitative arrangement of its parts there could be no individual bodies at all. This is why an individual body, however small, cannot be reduced to a mathematical point. The name given to the ultimate particle that was believed to be incapable of actual division was the *atom*. Advances in nuclear physics have shown how misleading this name eventually turned out to be.

While the parts of an individual are real in as much as they share in the existence of the whole individual, they do not have any separate actual existence unless they split from the whole. Actual existence belongs only to the whole individual. When an individual body (A) is split into the right and left sides, two new individuals are formed (A1 and A2). Prior to the splitting, the two sides do not exist as separate things, but merely as sides of the one whole individual that actually exists. We could say that before the split the right and left sides existed potentially as individuals. A molecule of water is an example of a true individual body, even if it is microscopic. It can disintegrate to give rise to atoms of hydrogen and oxygen. The molecule of water exists as a whole, while all its parts share in its actual existence. The parts themselves only exist potentially as separate beings. Hydrogen and oxygen can only come into actual existence when the molecule is split and loses its ontological individuality to give origin to new individuals, namely, atoms of hydrogen and oxygen.

The reverse may also occur. Hydrogen and oxygen atoms may interact and combine to form molecules of water. They are predisposed to react in this way to form water. But this does not mean that the form of water actually pre-exists to guide the process. When a spark is ignited, an explosion occurs during which the hydrogen and oxygen atoms lose their ontological individuality. This enables the form of water to arise from their matter to constitute new individual molecules of water. The notions of matter and form are introduced as real potential and actual principles of being, respectively, to explain this fundamental mutability demonstrated by material individuals. Each new individual has properties that simply cannot be explained by an artificial combination of parts. Form is required as an intrinsic principle of being to account for this new reality, i.e. water.

Material bodies either are individuals themselves or are composed of individuals that cohere closely together. They cannot exist in an indefinite, indeterminate or generic state. An individual body can only exist as a definite type of individual body, however small the particle. Each type of individual requires its own specific minimum quantity of matter, or mass, with a determinate structure or arrangement of its parts in order to exist. One need only think of the fixed atomic structure of the elements and compounds. Water needs to be formed from two atoms of hydrogen and one of oxygen arranged according to a definite pattern to constitute an actual individual molecule of water, even if they normally exist as pairs. The same applies, with all the more reason, for the more complex molecules. In the case of inorganic individuals any addition or subtraction of matter results in a change of kind of individual – i.e. a substantial change. Carbon monoxide gas is poisonous. The addition of one oxygen atom to each molecule of carbon monoxide changes it into non-poisonous carbon dioxide.

Viewed mathematically, individuals may be homogeneous. One could have a handful of identical diamonds and so speak of a collection of homogeneous diamonds. Within each individual diamond, however, not only are the parts distinct, they are heterogeneous. In other words at the atomic level, different parts display different structures and properties in the nuclear and electronic zones. The same applies within the individual molecule of water. Two of its regions resemble hydrogen while only one resembles oxygen in each individual molecule. In fact, we can attribute the potency of water to produce hydrogen and oxygen to this specifically determined molecular structure and arrangement of its quantitative parts. It appears that every individual must have heterogeneous parts if it is able to be divided at all. Unless this were the case, it would be hard to see how the necessary tension between at least two parts could arise before disintegration could take place.

Each type of individual has its own specific heterogeneous structure. This accounts for its nature, its properties and all its natural characteristics. The specific heterogeneity of the parts of an individual determine its potential for change once it disintegrates and loses its own ontological individuality. Because of its specific structure water only has the potency to break down into hydrogen and oxygen in the simplest of situations. The same applies when atoms of hydrogen and oxygen lose their individuality to become water. New individuals may arise from matter either by the combination or the dissolution of other individuals. In either case, new individuals can only begin if their respective forms are already potentially present in the matter of existing individuals in relation to their specific heterogeneous structure. This is why the results of chemical reactions between given individual substances or agents are not a chance affair. The forms that eventually actuate matter to constitute new individuals after chemical reactions are dependent on the previous potency of the matter from which they are derived. This is why human gametes can only produce human embryos, not sheep embryos – to cite a biological example.

Usually we succeed in identifying large individuals such as crystals and living individuals quite easily. Scientists can readily identify individuals at the atomic level and determine their structure. We should not, however, confuse the existence of distinct individuals, quite identifiable in principle, with our practical ability to distinguish them or pin-point their space–time co-ordinates. In some cases we might not know whether we had a separate individual or an aggregate of individuals. We could identify each grain of sand in a bucket, even if many were identical. The matter of one grain would not be that of another. They would be separate existent individuals even if in all other respects they were identical. The case would be different with grains of sand in concrete that has set. We might not be able to tell if we had one large individual piece of concrete or many individual grains tightly bound together. The test would be to see if they retained their chemical properties. A rod of iron encased in concrete would still be a rod of iron.

There is no reason why synthetic materials could not be genuine individuals. Complex molecules may be synthesized from atoms whether the process occurs naturally or not. It is a matter of seeing whether the compound behaves as one individual or many acting closely together. If a new property appears in the compound that cannot be explained by a mechanical combination of its constituent parts, it is a sign that a new individual has been formed. Maintenance of all individual functions and behaviour would indicate an aggregate with an artificial unity. The loss of independent functions and behaviour by the constituent parts would be a sign that they had lost their separate individuality and had merged to form one new individual with different properties and behaviour. A sandcastle on the beach would still be an aggregate of individual grains of sand with an artificial unity, but a piece of newly made glass would be a new distinct individual. For the purposes of ordinary living, it is of little importance to know whether a particular inorganic body is one genuine individual or many individuals closely knit together, giving only an appearance of ontological individuality. It is of paramount importance in the case of a mass of developing embryonic human cells.

One final refinement needs to be made to our understanding of an individual and its continuing ontological identity. Once a molecule comes into being and continues to exist uninterruptedly, it is the same ontological individual. If two molecules of water, x and y are changed into hydrogen and oxygen atoms through electrolysis, they cease to exist as the same ontological individuals. If the same hydrogen and oxygen atoms were again to be chemically changed into two molecules of water, they would form two new individual molecules of water, c and d, not x and y, even though they would be identical in every other respect. An individual's continuing ontological identity both requires, and is expressed in, continuous existence of the same body. The existence of the first pair would not be that of the second pair. This hypothetical example highlights the existential dimension of the meaning of an ontological individual retaining its identity in time.

9   The concept of a living ontological individual

It would be helpful to understand human individuals and their beginnings to consider briefly the specific nature of living individuals. What is true of inorganic individuals is, in general, also true of living individuals. These are usually easier to identify because they are big enough to see with the naked eye in most cases. The variations in their degrees of dynamic equilibrium and of natural unity suggests that the concept of *individual* is not *univocal* but *analogous*. What is to count as a living ontological individual will depend on the concept of individual that is employed. Each type of individual realizes its individuality in a different way. We believe the scientists when they tell us that each molecule has its specific heterogeneous quantitative parts corresponding to the characteristic arrangement of its constituent atoms. We can see for ourselves the specific heterogeneous structure of various living individuals like cats, dogs and humans. We can tell the difference between bones, flesh, organic tissues and blood.

Just as inorganic bodies are either individuals or are aggregates of individuals, so too living matter can be reduced to being the matter of living individuals. Living matter belongs to living individuals. In the case of a live organ that has been removed for transplantation, we could speak of it in a diminished sense of individuality. The organ was part of a living individual and could soon be integrated into another living individual after a successful transplant. If one wished to persist, one could still speak of living individual cells that retain some organic coherence until decay commences, in the absence of a successful transplant. Admittedly, our categories do break down somewhat in the case of decaying organic matter. Not all organs and tissues cease to be alive the instant death occurs in a human or other living individuals. When a living organism dies as a whole, the live organs and tissues only gradually disintegrate and lose life. Could this be a sign that perhaps at the outset, individual cells first form specific tissues, systems of cells and regions before the whole organism is constituted as an individual?

Molecules of water are not only of the same type of substance. They are identical, alike in every respect with exactly the same characteristics. The same is true of identical mammalian twins that originate from one fertilized egg when the proliferating cells divide into two masses of cells and develop independently. Just as the molecules of water are chemically identical, but not ontologically, so also identical twin organisms are genetically identical, but not ontologically identical. This is because they are two distinct individuals, not one. All molecules of water are chemically identical, but only those twins that derive from the same fertilized egg or embryo are genetically identical. If, as we shall see, identical twin mouse embryos were to be aggregated together to form one embryo again, while it would be genetically identical with the original parent mouse embryo, it could hardly be the same ontological individual mouse embryo. If, say, the original mouse embryo was named *Tom*, then the unnamed twins could not re-constitute *Tom* when they recombined but another mouse, say *Jerry*. These examples may be entertaining, but they serve to illustrate the implications of the concept of an ontological individual and its on-going ontological identity.

An individual, granted a favourable environment and suitable nourishment, in virtue of being alive, of its own power from within itself, actively strives to be self-maintaining, self-developing and functioning for its own welfare. This is the essence of being a living individual. If this life ceases definitively through a complete loss of potency for life, there is no longer a living individual present, but a corpse, deprived of its previous ontological identity. It is different if the life process of an individual has only been slowed down almost to the point of zero metabolic rate. A frozen embryo is not dead – it is still alive. Its metabolic rate only suffices to preserve its potential for sustaining life, not for development or growth. This represents a case of self-preservation or suspended animation while life is dormant. The live embryo that survives thawing is the same ontological embryo that underwent the freezing process. The frozen embryo is re-activated once it is thawed. The frozen embryo resembles a seed that may lie dormant for ages until it germinates when suitable environmental conditions prevail. On the other hand, a thoroughly roasted grain of wheat is not alive, having lost all inherent potency for further development and growth.

An inorganic individual normally comes into being instantaneously and rather completely, without any further potential for development or eventual reproduction. The existence of a living individual is spread out not only in space but also in time. Time is required for those activities that are self-maintaining and self-developing.[28] These activities continue until they perfect or complete the very being of the living individual throughout a period that is called its lifetime. Life is a process, a cycle during which this sort of inborn potential, characteristically determined for each species, is naturally realized for each individual. Living activities are immanent: they can only take place within the individual to realize its self-maintenance, self-development and growth. As long as it lives, an organic individual unceasingly actualizes its potential to remain in being without loss of ontological identity. Its grasp on existence is fragile and consequently it is mortal.

The same individual that begins life goes through its life-cycle. This involves considerable changes in the quantity of the matter possessed by each individual at various stages of life. One's identity as a living ontological individual remains unchanged whenever one gains or loses weight. The same is true if one loses one or more limbs.[29] One keeps one's own identity throughout several successful organ transplants. What is needed to remain the same ontological individual is to stay alive, sustained by the functioning of one's vital organs all the time. It is the form that actuates the matter to make it be a living individual of a specific species. (Remember the soul acts as form for the human individual.) The cells of one's body could be totally renewed over a period of six years without loss of one's individual ontological identity. As this gradually takes place, the new matter is integrated into the one existing living individual.

It is the individual as a whole that exists primarily, not the single cells. The cells and organs share in the life and existence of the whole individual. They do not exist separately or at least as distinct individuals themselves. (Exceptions do exist where some distinct individuals live within another living individual, e.g. sperm, ova, bacteria, viruses, the fetus in the mother's womb, the mother's protective white cells passed to the baby's gut during breast feeding.) The one living individual continues in existence throughout all the changes of its self-development and growth. Matter from outside the organism can be taken in and assimilated by the process of nutrition to become one with the same living ontological individual. Inorganic individuals cannot do this and lose their ontological identity if their atomic composition is altered, as we have seen already in the case of atoms and molecules. It is clear that the living organism assimilates from within to grow as the same ontological individual.[30] A living individual, however, should be understood analogously as eminently dynamic, fluid, and developmental, compared to its rigid inorganic counterpart.

John Locke saw quite clearly that human identity was tied to the human body and its continuing life-principle. A dualistic view of a soul separated from the human body could explain neither the continuity of identity of one man from the beginning nor of one distinct man among many. I can only agree with him when he argues as follows on the identity of man:

> This also shows wherein the identity of the same *man* consists; viz. in nothing but a participation of the same continued life, by constantly fleeting particles of matter, in succession vitally united to the same organized body. He that shall place the identity of man in anything else, but, like that of other animals, in one fitly organized body, taken in any one instant, and from thence continued, under one organization of life, in several successively fleeting particles of matter united to it, will find it hard to make an embryo, one of years, mad and sober, the *same* man, by any supposition, that will not make it possible for Seth, Ismael, Socrates, Pilate, St. Austin, and Caesar Borgia, to be the same man. For if the identity of *soul alone* makes the same *man*; and there be nothing in the nature of matter why the same individual spirit may not be united to different bodies, it will be possible that those men, living in distant ages, and of different tempers, may have been the same man: which way of speaking must be from a very strange use of the word man, applied to an idea out of which body and shape are excluded.[31]

It is the individual that is the subject of the life process and all its activities. Life is not independent of the individual that is alive. Nutrients might come from outside the organism, but nutrition itself takes place from within the individual to provide the energy needed to enable its living activities to proceed. The individual's heterogeneous quantitative parts share in its life by being organized and geared to contribute to the self-maintenance, self-development, growth, repair, and well-being of the one complex organism. All its parts, cells, structures, organization and activities are subordinated to serve its common interests and goals of life, directed by its species-specific instructions encoded in its programme of life.

The intrinsic directiveness of a living individual's activities for the achieving of set goals or purposes within the organism is quite distinct from how the goals of life are promoted by interactions and exchanges between various living individuals in the natural order of things. How would animals survive without grasses, plants and their fruits? Some animals naturally live by preying on others. Teleology within living individuals must not be confused with teleology between living individuals. This distinction is particularly relevant in the sphere of reproductive biology in mammals. Maternal functions and responses that facilitate the conception, implantation, growth and development of the fetus should not be mistaken for purely fetal activities of self-development and growth alone. The purposeful activities of interaction and cooperation between maternal and fetal tissues and organs show natural teleology at work *between* two living individuals rather than directive activities of a single individual organism, namely the mother. The activities of the mother that protect, support and sustain the fetus are essential, but they are not the living activities of the fetus itself.

It is crucial to bear in mind one additional distinction. The self-development of a living individual through its processes of cell multiplication and differentiation needs to be carefully distinguished from the formation of a new individual that results from the combination of individual cells or cell-systems endowed with the requisite developmental potential. It is not enough for the formation of a new individual to have many individual cells, be they haploid or diploid, that merely have the potential to fuse or aggregate together to become a new organism. A living individual, even though dormant, must be specifically determined and actually constituted with its own natural life-principle for it to begin to exist. The constituent cells would have to lose their own separate individuality before they became living heterogeneous parts contributing to the maintenance and welfare of a new living individual. Its life-principle would need to take precedence over, and subordinate to its own functioning, the activities of these same cells before a single organism could arise to incorporate them into being part of itself. This would be required for the presence of a living ontological individual with the retention of the same ontological identity throughout all its successive stages of development.

E. S. Russell was right in making the following points in explaining his concept of organism:

> Primary characteristics of the living organism are then the directive, creative and orderly nature of its activities in relation to maintenance, reproduction and development, to the completion of the normal life-cycle; primary conditions of existence are the preservation of structuro–functional wholeness or normality, and integral adaptation to an environment (or series of environments) in which the particular needs and requirements of the organism for the completion of its life-cycle can be satisfied.
>
> It is important to note that the conditions of existence must be *actively* established and maintained. Structuro–functional wholeness or integrity, and specific structure, are actively built up and maintained in the course of development, chiefly by the morphogenetic and behavioural activity of cells or groups of cells ... the organism strives to persist in its own being, and to reach its normal completion or actualisation. This striving is not as a rule a conscious one, nor is there often any foresight of the end, but it exists all the same, as the very core of the organism's being.[32]

10   A potential person

Frequently, reference is made to the notion of potential person in ordinary discourse as well as in Government Reports. It would be useful at this point to briefly analyse the various meanings the phrase *potential person* has in as much as they are relevant to our task.

A child is sometimes said to be a potentially great scholar, musician or footballer. In this sense the child is actually a human person with the inherent potential to mature or develop certain talents or skills. The child may be said to be the adult in the sense that he continues to be the same actual person throughout, but actually acquires in time what was only previously present potentially (e.g. adulthood). This inherent potential for development is to be distinguished from the potential to receive an extrinsic entitlement, e.g. the right to accession to the throne of the United Kingdom. We may say Prince Charles is potentially the King of England in accordance with the law of succession. We shall not be concerned with these instances of potentiality because in both cases an *actual* human person already exists.

It is interesting to observe that life in a living individual represents a special characteristic, a perfection or actuality, in comparison to non-living individuals. Yet life itself, while being an actual characteristic, is at one and the same time itself potential, i.e. it has the inherent active potency for further life. To be alive means to live on, to be living, to have the potential for further living. Life is not a static reality. Life represents something dynamic in an entity whereby it strives to hold onto further existence precisely by living. A dead individual has lost its potential or capacity to prolong its existence or being. To kill a human being means to deprive an individual of the potential to live on and to make free choices that may influence one's ultimate destiny. Loss of such potential is the loss of life and the cessation of a human individual in the world of our experience. To be a living person means one still has the active potential for further development and growth or at least survival as a being.

It is becoming increasingly obvious that potentiality or potency is an analogous notion, whose meaning may be somewhat elastic, referring to various degrees of real potency to actuality – from remote to proximate. Potentiality is correlative to actuality. At times it is said that the sperm or the egg is a potential person. We know neither one is an actual person, but through the process of successful fertilization, both together may give rise to an actual person, immediately, or after some development. This is all that can be meant by referring to one or the other as a potential person – indeed, merely a remotely potential person. In the natural state and in the absence of fertilization, neither taken separately nor jointly do they have any inherent active potential to form a person. This is a crucial difference. Indeed, they have very little potential for further life if fertilization does not intervene. It is quite misleading to refer to sperm or egg in themselves as a potential person except in a very weak sense of the term. Taken separately, but considered jointly, they are not the same ontological entity as the single-cell zygote that results from their fusion and which may be said to be a potential person. They should not be considered to be a potential person in the same sense because they are different kinds of entity or types of individual living being.[33] Quite rightly, independent moral protection is not generally accorded to the human sperm or egg, whereas it should be given to the human zygote after the gametes join to form a new cell.

Once fertilization has taken place the human sperm and egg cease to exist as distinct entities. A genetically human, new living individual cell is formed, a zygote, that has the proximate potential to become a mature human person with the same genetic constitution. While many regard the zygote as a human person already in its own right, others, but not all, regard it as a potential person, i.e. as an entity with the inherent active potential to become a human person, given favourable conditions. The Warnock Report unanimously:

> ...agreed that the embryo of the human species ought to have a special status and that ... the embryo of the human species should be afforded some protection in law.[34]

In a minority expression of dissent it was argued that though the early embryo was not yet a person, similar respect was due to it:

> ...the embryo has a special status because of its potential for development to a stage at which everyone would accord it the status of a person. It is in our view wrong to create something with the potential for becoming a person and then deliberately to destroy it.[35]

While all members of the Warnock Committee agreed some respect should be shown to the human embryo, the minority argued this respect should be absolute. This is based on the inherent developmental potential of the embryo, already possessed of genetically human life, to become a human individual. Though this is not the place to develop a moral treatise, the practical significance of a human embryo as a potential person cannot be divorced from certain moral considerations and principles to which I must briefly allude.

Nobody suggests that the development of a mouse embryo ought not be impeded. It is not simply the impeding of the development of life of any, or every, embryo that is the crux of the moral problem. The case of the human embryo is different in this respect for several reasons, even if it is considered only as a potential person. Its moral significance is derived from the fact that it is the fruit of human generation, derived from the gametes of human parents. It is already endowed with genetically human life that is naturally destined to become a human person, given a suitable maternal environment for normal development. The purpose or finality of the human procreative process ought not be rendered void by preventing the human embryo becoming an actual personal being. The procreative process is undertaken for the sake of a new human individual in whom its meaning is realized. Lack of respect shown to a human embryo flouts our own personal dignity as well as that of the embryonic future person (if development is allowed to get that far). For the believer, the duty to respect human embryos is reinforced by the conviction that the divine plan for the responsible transmission of human life as the fruit of conjugal love should never be deliberately frustrated. From fertilization onwards, genetically human life is to be fostered as God's gift.

The duty to protect human embryos becomes clearer the closer they approach in their development to becoming truly human persons in actuality. It is a sign of our humanness that we instinctively feel more repelled from harming embryos as their developmental process brings them closer to sharing in our common dignity and natural, if not legal, personhood. We owe it to our humanity to respect not only persons, but also the biologically human life of cells that, in this hypothesis, are destined soon to become human individuals. Human persons come into existence through genetically human life. Whatever has human life is closely related to human beings and thereby acquires a special moral significance. Baroness Warnock echoed this basic moral intutition when she wrote:

> It is part of our humanity that we should regard fellow members of the species as in a special relation to ourselves.[36]

She stops short of requiring absolute respect for the human embryo, whereas others insist on absolute protection for an embryo considered as a potential person principally on account of the human significance of its genetically human life and its unique relationships to the plan of the Creator as Lord and Giver of Life. At the end of life, we do respect a human corpse precisely because it once was a living human person. Rather than speak of the rights of a corpse, we view our obligations towards a corpse as flowing from a need to respect our own innate sense of human dignity.

I believe the meaning of a potential person needs to be understood in the context of genetically human life and of the above moral concepts. While the wilful killing of a human individual, gifted by the Creator with an opportunity to choose a happy eternal destiny, is homicide, the deliberate destruction of a potential person would, by reason of its biologically human life, be immoral, but not technically homicide. There is a challenge for moralists as well as lawyers and embryologists to invent new terms as we all come to grips with new cases and situations that involve the care, treatment and possible disposal of embryonic human life.

11   The task ahead

After these preliminary discussions on the concept of a developing human individual, the criteria for determining its beginning and the concepts of both inorganic and living individuals, we are better equipped to take up the challenge of seeking an answer to the question of when a human individual begins. We cannot draw *a priori* conclusions in this regard without a detailed examination of the relevant biological facts of human reproduction. All the available evidence needs to be considered in the light of philosophical concepts and metaphysical principles that are both intelligible and adequate for the task.

It is a matter of determining when a distinct living individual is first formed that has the natural active potential to begin the continuous process of developing itself into an adult human individual while retaining throughout its own ontological identity as a living individual. It is necessary to differentiate between the potential of proliferating cells to become a human individual and the potential of a human individual to develop itself and grow through the multiplication and differentiation of its cells. It is a matter of determining whether the early human embryo is one human individual or many individual cells. It is a matter of tracing the typical ontological identity of a distinct adult human individual back as far as possible to its beginning as a distinct living human individual. It is necessary to assess the effects of the phenomenon of identical twinning in human embryos on the presence of a continuing ontological identity in the human individuals concerned. The same is to be said of the possibility of identical twinning and not only of actual identical twinning.

There is no telling in advance the minimum specific mass or number of cells required for the origin of a distinct human individual from fertilization onwards. This is something to be noted. Variations may occur in this respect in relation to the developmental stage achieved by the human embryonic cells concerned in the case of twinning. This would not be surprising for the quantitative parts of a human individual are the bearers of its specific qualitative heterogeneity in which the individual's processes of life unfold. The quantitative aspects of a living individual should not be interpreted statically. The quantitative dimension is totally caught up with the life processes of an individual from the outset. The quantitative features of a human individual cannot be divorced from the dynamism of its life any more than its life processes can be taken independently of its specific quantitative requirements. Consideration should be given to both factors when discerning the beginning of the living human individual.

It now remains to see if the human individual begins at fertilization, retaining the same individual ontological identity until adulthood through self-development and growth. If this proves to be inconclusive, it will be necessary to consider further stages of development of the human embryo to see if there is sufficient evidence at any other particular point of development to positively establish when the human individual begins, or before which this could not occur, or probably could not occur. Although I am satisfied that the human individual is a person, there certainly could not be a person if there could not be an ontological individual formed before any particular stage of human biological development.[37] An ongoing ontological individual that retains its identity and is biologically human marks the beginning of human personhood, but not the end of personal development. This continues throughout one's whole life, influenced by one's family, education, religion, culture and most of all by one's free choices.

4

Fertilization and the beginning of a human individual

Having established that a human being must be both an ontological individual and a living ontological individual, it now remains to reflect philosophically on the relevant scientific evidence to determine when these two criteria are first satisfied in the species *Homo sapiens*. It would be wise to begin with a brief review of the pertinent biological facts from fertilization onwards. There is broad agreement amongst embryologists concerning these facts. Disagreements arise among both biologists and philosophers when it comes to interpreting the scientific data in relation to the beginning of a new human individual.

1   Fertilization

At fertilization there begins a new, genetically unique, living individual, when the sperm and the ovum lose their separate individualities to form a single living cell, a zygote. Fertilization is not a momentary event but a process that may last up to 20–24 hours, beginning with the first contact of the sperm with the plasma membrane of the secondary oocyte (ovum) and finishing with the mixing of the maternal and paternal chromosomes (syngamy) to constitute the zygote. After the process of fertilization is completed the ovum becomes the single–cell pre-implanted zygote prior to its first mitotic division (cleavage) into two smaller identical daughter cells.[1] The term 'zygote' is sometimes used to refer to the product of conception for a few days or even a fortnight. In this book I shall use 'zygote' to refer only to the diploid cell that results from the completion of fertilization.

Each spermatozoon and ovum is an individual, a living cell, distinct from the mother and father. In due time, these separate individuals fuse to form the fertilized ovum. This is called the zygote because it yokes together the maternal and paternal genetic contributions for the formation of a new living cell. It is also an individual organism, quite distinct from the sperm and egg from which it is derived. It is not a simple cell at all, but an extremely complex structure with a hive of co-ordinated activities. Enclosed within the cell membrane are the nucleus and the cytoplasm. The nucleus is the centre of control for replicating DNA between cell cycles. In the cytoplasm proteins are synthesized, nutrients are conserved and activities occur in various tiny organs called organelles. These subcellular organelles are the mitochondria, the lysosomes, the ribosomes, the endoplasmic reticulum, the Golgi apparatus and the macromolecules of fats, carbohydrates, nucleic acids and proteins – to mention a few. They all play their role in the development of the embryo.

Each cell of the human body normally has 46 chromosomes (diploid), 23 sets of distinct maternal and paternal pairs, along which are located the genes that control the unique hereditary traits and characteristics of each individual. Except in the case of identical twins, they ensure that one individual does not closely resemble another. This is achieved in the following manner. During the formation of the sperm and the ovum (gametogenesis), the number of chromosomes in each germ cell is halved from 46 to 23 through a process called meiosis (first meiotic division) (see Fig. 4.1). During this process homologous maternal and paternal chromosomes split longitudinally, come together and may exchange regions of themselves by a mechanism known as 'crossing over'. They then separate and randomly segregate into two daughter cells such that each cell normally contains 23 distinct chromosomes, each of which is composed of a pair of chromatid threads and may be maternal or paternal in origin. 'Crossing over' and random segregation usually make these cells maternal/paternal composites. In this way the first meiotic division guarantees that each egg and sperm is genetically unique as a result of this random mix of genetic material. At meiosis in the oocyte one daughter cell always receives much less cytoplasm than the other and is normally extruded as the first polar body which eventually degenerates. The second meiotic division in spermiogenesis leaves each sperm with 23 chromosomes, each consisting of a single chromatid thread.

It is estimated that sperm may reach the egg in the fallopian tube any time between five and 68 minutes after coitus.[2] Sperm need a few hours to undergo various physiological changes in the female reproductive tract before they are able to penetrate the zona pellucida of the oocyte. These changes, known as capacitation and the acrosome reaction, precede penetration of the zona pellucida of the egg by the sperm (see Fig. 4.2).

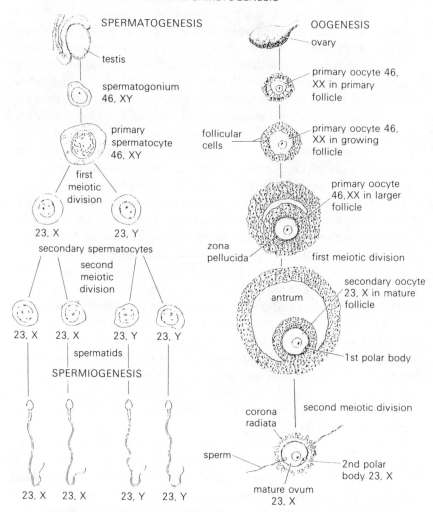

Fig. 4.1. Drawings comparing spermatogenesis and oogenesis. Oogonia are not shown in this diagram because all oogonia differentiate into primary oocytes before birth. The chromosome complement of the germ cells is shown at each stage. The number designates the total number of chromosomes, including the sex chromosome(s) shown after the comma. Note that (1) following the two meiotic divisions, the diploid number of chromosomes, 46, is reduced to the haploid number, 23; (2) *four sperms* form from one primary spermatocyte, whereas only *one* mature ovum results from maturation of a primary oocyte; and (3) the cytoplasm is conserved during oogenesis to form one large cell, the mature oocyte or ovum. (From K. Moore, *The Developing Human: Clinically Oriented Embryology*, Philadelphia: W. B. Saunders, 3rd edn, 1982, with slight modifications from colour to black and white.)

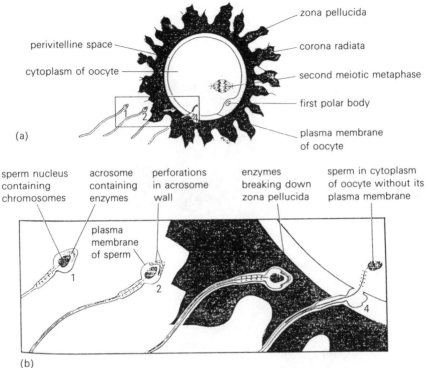

sperm nucleus containing chromosomes

acrosome containing enzymes

perforations in acrosome wall

enzymes breaking down zona pellucida

sperm in cytoplasm of oocyte without its plasma membrane

Fig. 4.2. Diagrams illustrating the acrosome reaction and sperm penetration of an oocyte. The detail of the area outlined in (*a*) is given in (*b*). *1*, Sperm during capacitation. *2*, Sperm undergoing the acrosome reaction. *3*, Sperm digesting a path through the zona pellucida by the action of enzymes released from the acrosome. *4*, Sperm after entering the cytoplasm of the oocyte. Note that (1) the plasma membranes of the sperm and the oocyte have fused, and (2) the head and tail of the sperm enter the oocyte, leaving the sperm's plasma membrane attached to the oocyte's plasma membrane. (From K. Moore, *The Developing Human: Clinically Oriented Embryology*, Philadelphia: W. B. Saunders, 3rd edn, 1982, with slight modifications from colour to black and white.)

The entry of the sperm into the ooplasm activates the oocyte to complete its second meiotic division, already begun at ovulation, and to extrude 23 chromosomes in the second polar body some 30–60 minutes later. The nuclei of both gametes are now haploid with 23 genetically unique chromosomes, each consisting of a single chromatid. Over the next few hours the sperm head decondenses and forms the male pronucleus inside its own nuclear envelope, while a membrane forms round the remaining 23 female chromosomes to form the female pronucleus. While they gradually move towards each other over the next 6–10 hours DNA synthesis takes place

FERTILIZATION

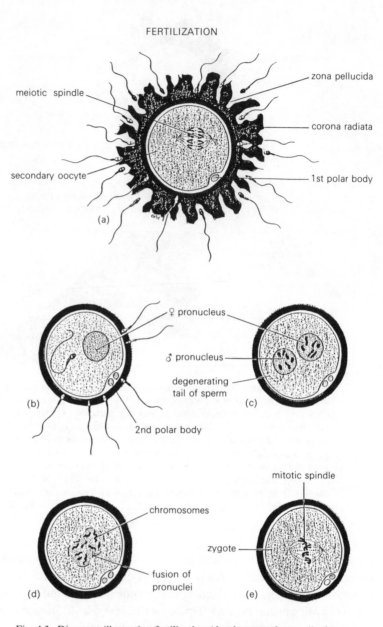

Fig. 4.3. Diagrams illustrating fertilization (developmental stage 1), the procession of events beginning when the sperm contacts the secondary oocyte's plasma membrane and ending with the intermingling of maternal and paternal chromosomes at metaphase of the first mitotic division of the zygote.
(*a*) Secondary oocyte surrounded by several sperms. (Only four of the 23 chromosome pairs are shown.) (*b*) The corona radiata has disappeared; a sperm

resulting in each chromosome becoming two identical chromatids (see Fig. 4.3). The pronuclei may be readily identified 12–18 hours after insemination during *in vitro* fertilization. According to Dr A. H. Sathananthan syngamy occurs about 22 hours after insemination when the membranes of the pronuclei break down about 6 hours after they are apposed, allowing the male and female chromosomes to mingle (personal communication). This marks the completion of fertilization and the constitution of the zygote, a single diploid cell with its own unique genotype. Its 23 pairs of homologous chromosomes soon pair up on the metaphase plate for the first mitotic cleavage about 24 hours after insemination.[3] Each homologous pair consists of one chromosome contributed by the father, and the other by the mother. Thus the genetic constitution of the new individual is established.

With the constitution of the individual's complete unique genetic package and gene pool during fertilization, the future development, growth and traits of the offspring are to a great extent, but not entirely, already practically determined. A reservation is mentioned because some traits, including build and height, are influenced by interactions between the genetic constitution and environment of the developing embryo and fetus. This implies the mother's health and uterine conditions have a great influence on the development of the child before birth in addition to general environmental factors throughout life after birth. The offspring's sex, however, is chromosomally determined at fertilization since the sex chromosome of the sperm has an almost equal probability of being male Y or female X. The sex chromosome of the egg is always female X so that a pair of XX chromosomes in the single-cell zygote produces female offspring, while an XY combination makes a male. Even so, external sexual differentiation does not begin to appear until many weeks later in embryonic development (see Appendix III).

Neither sperm nor egg alone without the other can give rise to a human baby. Through some accidents in nature the ovum may occasionally develop parthenogenetically without being fertilized by a sperm, before degenerating and dying during gestation. There is no proven case of a virgin birth in mammals. Normally only one sperm penetrates the zona

---

Caption for fig. 4.3 (*cont.*)

has entered the oocyte, and the second meiotic division has occurred, forming a *mature ovum*. (*c*) The sperm head has enlarged to form the male pronucleus. (*d*) The pronuclei are fusing. (*e*) The chromosomes of the zygote are arranged on a mitotic spindle in preparation for the first cleavage (mitotic) division. (From K. Moore, *The Developing Human: Clinically Oriented Embryology*, Philadelphia: W. B. Saunders, 3rd edn, 1982.)

pellucida containing the egg or secondary oocyte to fertilize it. This is due to a zona reaction after penetration by a sperm that renders the ovum impenetrable to any other sperm. Embryos that occasionally result from the fertilization of an egg by more than one sperm nucleus are not viable and usually abort spontaneously shortly afterwards or die soon after birth. The same can be said about some congenitally defective embryos with more or less than the normal 46 chromosomes due to the formation of chromosomally abnormal gametes during disjunction in their first or second meiotic divisions.

The most important macromolecules in the nucleus are the deoxyribonucleic acids (DNA), responsible ultimately for programming the specific activities of protein synthesis and development of cells. When a gene is activated a copy of the relevant section of DNA is made in ribonucleic acid (RNA) called a primary transcript. This is further processed in the nucleus before moving to the cytoplasm as messenger RNA to direct the synthesis of the relevant proteins by the ribosomes. The DNA is a template for the primary RNA transcript and eventual messenger RNA. Only a small stretch of DNA or gene is used in each cell. The part of the DNA thread that is selected for use determines the activities of that cell at any one time. Each cell of the human body from the zygote to adult stage contains all the genes of a human individual. It is the selective activation of genes that accounts for cell specialization.[4]

The unicellular zygote has many heterogeneous parts, but it is not an aggregate of distinct parts as though each part existed separately resulting in the formation of an aggregate or artificial unity. Notwithstanding dependence on the mother for survival, it shows all the signs of a single living individual since its activities are all directed from within in an orderly fashion for its self-maintenance and eventual cleavage into two smaller identical daughter cells through the process of mitosis. It harnesses the energies of atoms and molecules in determinate structures for its own life processes, self-development and well-being. The point of entry of the sperm in the mammalian egg has no significance for determining the embryo's axes of symmetry for its subsequent development. Human, and mammalian zygotes in general, do not resemble amphibian zygotes in this respect. Early mammalian embryos from the zygote stage show no symmetry in development, except for radial symmetry.

2   The case for a human individual beginning at fertilization

There does not seem to be any controversy about the scientific facts involved in the process of fertilization. The same cannot be said about their significance in relation to the beginning of a human individual in the product of fertilization, namely, a single-cell zygote. In this section I shall present other people's arguments in favour of the human individual beginning at least from the completion of fertilization. In the following section I shall give my views and argue against their conclusions.

Undoubtedly the completion of the process of fertilization of the two haploid germ cells to give a diploid single-cell zygote that is genetically determined for the whole development of its future life process is of capital importance. This is why fertilization is generally thought to constitute the beginning of a living individual human being that is ontologically unique. Except in the case of monozygotic twins, it is genetically unique as well. The genetic information encoded in the DNA of the genes and chromosomes of the fertilized ovum programmes, controls and co-ordinates its systematic development and integrated differentiation into various types of cells, tissues, structures, organs and limbs throughout the entire life process from fertilization onwards. Given suitable conditions and the right environment in the mother's body, together with an adequate supply of the proper nutrients, it seems that the same single-cell zygote, through multiple cleavages, development and growth alone, normally becomes a fetus, an infant, a child and an adult. It appears to be the very same individual living being from fertilization that has the inborn active potentiality to organize its own growth and self-development. The zygote is a distinct entity, with respect to its mother from the beginning, even though it does depend on her for survival, support, growth. This dependence on the mother, and others as well, continues for some years after birth, though to a lesser extent and in quite different ways. It is autonomous, however, in relation to the genetic information required for programming its orderly development. The zygote and the adult that develops from it have the same genetic individuality or identity.

The embryo from the outset has the inherent natural active capacity to direct and organize its own self-maintenance and self-development in relation to the structures and functions of its various parts, tissues and organs. This apparently occurs within the unity of a single multicellular human organism that continues to grow to the adult stage with the very same ontological identity from the single-cell zygote stage. This seems to be the start of individuation. This is when the genetic components of ovum and sperm become one to form a highly complex and centrally organized individual cell, endowed with its own genetic and ontological individuality that appears to endure throughout subsequent development.

An individual ovum and an individual sperm fuse to form a new distinct living individual.

The fertilized ovum must not be thought of as a tiny human being, complete with all its organs, that only needs to grow to become an adult. Preformation with its 'homunculus', once believed to reside in the spermhead or ovum, has long been rejected by all biologists. Instead, the zygote develops epigenetically in the sense of having all the sufficient and necessary genetic information contained within itself, together with the active power to organize and build itself up from this tiny cell. As though it were a miniature computer selecting and following its own internal programme, it seems to actuate its own inherent potential through the life processes of a single developing human individual. Robert Edwards seems to agree when, referring to the fertilized ovum as it divides:

> It becomes magnificently organized, switching on its own bio-chemistry, increasing in size, and preparing itself quickly for implantation in the womb.[5]

There are good reasons for believing the same ontological identity is retained throughout every stage of growth and development of the human person from fertilization. In fact, fertilization is the most biologically significant stage in the whole process of the transmission of human life. There does not appear to be any other comparable discontinuity in the process of reproduction to warrant settling on any other stage to mark the beginning of the life of an individual human being. The mitotic cleavages and multiplication of cells from fertilization onwards continue without any apparent prejudice to the unity and continuity of existence of the same ontological individual in the zygote, the multicellular embryo, the fetus, the infant, the child and the adult person.

In this regard we need to distinguish between passive and active potentiality. Hydrogen and oxygen have the passive potentiality to combine to form water but they are not yet actually water. The same can be said of the sperm and ovum. They have the passive potentiality to fuse and become a zygote but taken separately they are not actually a zygote and cannot become one if they remain apart. There appear to be good reasons to believe that the zygote itself already is an actual human being with the active potential for self-directive development until the ability to exercise intelligent and free activity is acquired, and beyond.

It seems logical that personhood could not be conferred from without at some subsequent stage if the inherent potential for truly human development were not already present in the zygote. Surely this intrinsic active potentiality for development to human adulthood could only be possessed by a living ontological individual with a truly human nature. The human zygote should be considered a human individual, so the argument goes, because it has the same nature and ontological identity as the adult that is derived from it by growth and development. Relating to other persons through a variety of personal contacts, from infancy onwards, helps one enormously to express better one's personhood and to develop psychologically and socially. All this, however, presupposes the presence of personhood but it does not constitute it. The human zygote cannot grow into anything but a human being.

Once a human individual begins to exist, changes in the size and the material elements in the make-up of the human individual during the period of growth do not change its ontological identity. The new material elements are absorbed, assimilated and integrated into one underlying unified organic system as living parts of the human person that continues its existence substantially unchanged as an ontological individual. It is the same individual human being from the zygote stage onwards that, by virtue of its natural dynamic capacity, transforms itself through growth and self-development with its genetic, biological and psychosomatic unity and identity unchanged. Continuity of genetic identity of the zygote with the subsequent adult would, it is held, strongly support the ontological and personal identity of the zygote and the human individual that develops from it.

The unicellular zygote, with its specific heterogeneous quantitative parts characteristically arranged, seems to have the minimum mass of living matter required for the constitution of an ontological individual with a truly human nature. It is thought to be a human individual because it is assumed to have the natural capacity to develop to human adulthood without loss of its ontological individuality. In short, it is argued that from the completion of fertilization (syngamy) we have a human being or person with potential, not a potential human person. It would appear the criteria for being a human individual established in the previous chapter point to this conclusion beyond reasonable doubt. The adult, then, would be the same personal being as the zygote from which it develops through cell multiplication, differentiation and growth.

A difficulty is raised by R. Edwards and J. Diamond against the view that the human individual begins at the zygote stage on account of the phenomenon of identical twinning.[6] They doubt whether it is possible for the zygote to be a human individual if it can give rise subsequently to two identical daughter cells that may develop separately and be born as identical twins. More precisely, it is claimed, one human individual cannot give rise to two distinct human individuals without dying or losing its own individuality. It would be hard to admit the presence of an individual human being in the zygote if, in principle, it could lose its ontological identity whenever twinning occurs in the course of development.

One answer often given to this difficulty is drawn from the experience of gardeners. A slip from some plants may be cut and planted in the soil to give rise to a new plant without the original plant dying or ceasing to be the same living individual. Here one living individual gives origin to another individual without losing its own individual existence. A human person may produce new individuals without loss of ontological identity quite frequently in life – sperm and ova are special distinct living individuals, even if they can only survive for a day or so in normal circumstances! Another theoretical answer would be to allow that upon twinning, two new individuals arise with the original human individual ceasing to exist at the zygote stage. Such an explanation of asexual generation of identical twins might not be appealing, but it is theoretically conceivable. Hence, it is argued, the mere fact of, or even the possibility of, the zygote giving origin to one or more distinct individuals does not in theory prove there could not have been a single individual in the first place. Think of how a bacterial cell becomes two cells by binary fission. One *organism* may give origin to *two organisms*. In the same way could not one human individual give origin to two? This means the human zygote could *actually* be one human individual, but *potentially* two.

T. V. Daly, a Jesuit priest, *summarily* answers the thrust of the difficulty posed by identical twinning in the following passage, which was also included in evidence submitted to the Australian Parliament's *Senate Select Committee on the Human Embryo Experimentation Bill 1985*:

> There is nothing philosophically troublesome about one organized whole developing within it another circle of organization which eventually breaks off from it while the original individual retains its identity. One living thing has given rise to another and this can happen in a wide variety of ways, most of which are quite familiar, though so many writers on the embryo assume that this would destroy all previous individuality. The twinning that they see as an unsuperable (*sic*) obstacle to previous establishment of identity is no more difficult to explain than is the vegetative propagation of a plant by removing a bulb, or by taking a cutting. An amoeba is no less of a real concrete individual living thing if later on it reproduces and initiates a new

amoeba by fission. Indeed the same applies for sexual reproduction. If we were to take seriously the line of argument of Diamond, Edwards and the like, we would have to deny that a man or a woman had ever been an individual once we found that he or she had produced a child.[7]

It is well known that maternally derived messenger RNA in the cytoplasm of the ovum controls development of the zygote at least up to the two-cell stage, before which time the embryo's genes have not yet been expressed or its genome 'switched-on' genetically. This would be consistent with the absence of RNA synthesis during fertilization. Until this occurs the early embryo only utilizes gene products synthesized during oogenesis and stored in the egg. This genetic silence lasts all during egg maturation, fertilization and possibly up to the four-cell stage in humans, when the embryo's own genotype gradually assumes complete control of development. During this period the maternal RNA progressively degenerates.[8] These facts suggest that perhaps the zygote should not be regarded as a human individual if the newly established genotype is not in control of the early stages of development. Daly dismisses this objection rather summarily, pointing out that this information:

> ...is perfectly compatible with the fact that a distinct new individual is established at fertilization, since it is obvious that the cytoplasm need not cease making a contribution within the new cell, and the main 'changes' and 'activity' at this stage and until the formation of the blastula concern the synthesis and replication of DNA to provide for all the cell multiplications. This DNA, which is the centre of the activity, is, of course, that with the new genome, formed by equal contributions from the paternal and maternal germ cells.[9]

Once it is admitted that the zygote represents the beginning of the development of the human individual, the same unicellular individual becomes a multicellular individual without loss of ontological individuality. The development and growth of the human individual through mitotic proliferation of cells and differentiation inevitably involves some cell movement and even migration of cells. In itself this should not present any insuperable problems for the continuity of existence of the same ontological living individual since this occurs quite normally in the human adult. Think of the movement of blood cells, hormones, enzymes, etc., in a normally functioning human body. Considerable self-regulated movement of cells is also involved in the repair of tissues during the healing of wounds, be they internal or superficial without prejudice to the continuing ontological identity of a human individual.

The same individual continues to exist notwithstanding the successful transplanting of vital organs such as the heart or kidney from another donor human individual. Once the newly transplanted organ *takes* and becomes integrated into the living structure of the recipient human individual, it loses whatever separate residual organic individuality it still possessed. It becomes a part of another living human individual that absorbs it without detriment to its own continuing ontological identity. In a similar way a developing early human embryo could assimilate into itself cells aggregated to it from one or more other early human embryos to become a human chimaera without loss of its own original ontological identity. Being a living individual does not exclude the assimilation of extraneous live tissue.

> ...a new centrally organized unity has been established, quite distinct from the organization of the preceding sperm or egg or mother cell, the genetic code of this new individual has been determined and a whole set of very remarkable capacities has been established. Allowing for the normal availability of nourishment and a non-hostile environment, that progenitor cell already has the capacity for directing its own development in such a way that a brain is developed suitable for all those activities which we saw to be characteristic of human beings, the activities that persons can perform. Those capacities already exist in the genetic material of the progenitor cell ... The fertilized cell is a new human person.[10]

These views are supported by B. M. Ashley, a Dominican priest:

> ...we now know that from the moment of perfect fertilization, the embryo develops through a principle intrinsic to it, namely, the genetic code contained in the primordial nucleus, and later, through the 'primary organizer' which appears in the blastocyst and then ultimately through the central nervous system. This genetic code embodied in this central organ in its various phases of development is not a mere 'blueprint', but also (and this is the essential point) a vital capacity to develop the whole organism into a mature human being, and it is this capacity for organic self-development into what is phenotypically a human person that we call the human-life principle or human soul.[11]

T. W. Hilgers, M.D., is more strongly supportive though he offers no philosophical reasons for his convictions:

> Once conception has occurred, an individual human life has come into existence and is a progressive, ongoing continuum until natural or artificially induced death ensues. This is a fact so well established within the reproductive sciences that no intellectually honest physician in full command of modern knowledge could dare to deny it. There is no authority in medicine or biology who can be cited to refute this concept.[12]

Quite authoritative backing comes from the finding of the *New Zealand Royal Commission of Inquiry into Contraception, Sterilization and Abortion*, 1977:

> From a biological point of view there is no argument as to when life begins. Evidence was given to us by eminent scientists from all over the world. None of them suggested that human life begins at any time other than at conception.[13]

Many other philosophers would agree with the commonly accepted general line of the argument that I have presented in favour of fertilization as the beginning of a new human being.[14] Most embryologists and biologists would appear to agree. The following passages from Keith Moore seem to confirm that the zygote marks the beginning of a human individual:

> Zygote. This cell results from fertilization of an oocyte, or ovum, by a sperm or spermatozoon, and is *the beginning of a human being*. The expression 'fertilized ovum' refers to the zygote.

> *Human development begins at fertilization*, when a sperm unites with an ovum to form a unicellular organism called a zygote (Gr. *zygotos*, yoked together). This cell marks the *beginnings* of each of us as a unique individual.[15]

Roberts, as well as Simpson and Beck express the same thought in their respective books:

> A human being originates in the union of two *gametes*, the ovum and the spermatozoon.[16]

> The fertilized egg cell – or zygote – contains nuclear material from both parents. It marks the beginning of the life of a new human being and is a useful focal point for presenting all the diverse aspects of organic reproduction.[17]

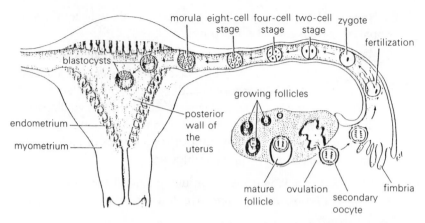

Fig. 4.4. Diagrammatic summary of the ovarian cycle, fertilization, and human development during the first week. Developmental stage 1 begins with fertilization and ends when the zygote forms. Stage 2 (days 2 to 3) comprises the early stages of cleavage (from 2 to about 16 cells or the morula). Stage 3 (days 4 to 5) consists of the free unattached blastocyst. Stage 4 (days 5 to 6) is represented by the blastocyst attaching to the centre of the posterior wall of the uterus, the usual site of implantation. (From K. Moore, *The Developing Human: Clinically Oriented Embryology*, Philadelphia: W. B. Saunders, 3rd edn, 1982.)

Finally, Hamilton and Mossman along with Patten concur:

Bisexual reproduction is characteristic of all vertebrates, and gametogenesis (the production of germ cells) is its first phase. The next phase, the beginning of the development of a new individual, is the fusion of two germ cells (gametes) of different nature; one, the spermatozoon from the male parent; the other, the ovum from the female parent. The result of this fusion is the formation of the first cell of the new individual, the zygote.[18]

The growth, the maturation, and all the factors leading toward the meeting of the male and female sex cells are but preliminary to their actual fusion. It is the penetration of the ovum by a spermatozoon and the resultant mingling of the nuclear material each brings to the union that constitutes the culmination of the process of fertilization and marks the initiation of the life of a new individual.[19]

3   The case against a human individual beginning at fertilization

The significance of fertilization in terms of the beginning of a new human individual is best understood in the light of what follows the completion of this process. In the first few days after fertilization the zygote within its protective shell cleaves into two equal cells, then four, eight, sixteen, etc. Mitotic division multiplies them as well as gradually reducing them to the size of normal somatic cells. They form a morula, a mulberry-like cluster of about 16 cells by the third day. They begin to form a blastocyst from the fourth day as entry is made to the uterus (see Fig. 4.4) prior to beginning the process of implantation, from about day seven to day 13 after fertilization. Saving mishaps, each cell contains the full complement of 23 pairs of maternal and paternal chromosomes – 46 in all. 42 cleavage divisions suffice to provide the billions of cells required for a baby at birth, while only another five divisions are required to reach the adult stage of the human individual.[20] Cell differentiation is quite pronounced after the first six cleavages and continues during the embryonic and fetal development stages of growth. This enables the various structures and organs to develop in order and harmony.

(i)   *Genetic and ontological individuality*

It is necessary to clearly distinguish between the concept of genetic and ontological individuality or identity. Biologists speak about one's genetic or biological identity or genome being established at fertilization. This is unique for each individual. Except in the case of identical twins, no two persons have the same genetic constitution or genotype. All the cells that derive from a single zygote have the same genetic make-up. This includes the cells that constitute the extra-embryonic membranes, placental tissues as well as the definitive embryo, fetus and adult. This is all that biologists mean when they say that genetic or biological individuality is established at fertilization. They are not speaking philosophically about the concept of a continuing ontological individual. No doubt some biologists, like many others in the community, could quite easily and uncritically take for granted that the human person also begins when genetic individuality is established. The existence of identical twins shows that genetic and ontological identity or individuality are not equivalent. The genetic code in the zygote does not suffice to constitute or define a human individual in an ontological sense. Identical twins have the same genetic code but they are distinct ontological individuals. Failure to appreciate this significant distinction could lead to a mistake in determining the timing of establishing the beginning of a human person.

It is interesting to note that a 'chorionic biopsy' can now be performed on the extraembryonic membrane tissue of the chorion to detect genetic diseases of the fetus itself. This is so because its genetic constitution is identical to that of the fetus. It is hoped to perfect this technique so that it may be used eventually without risk to the fetus or mother. In this case, one could scarcely argue that the subject of the biopsy was the human individual rather than chorionic tissue that has no nerves.

As we saw above, the embryonic genome is not switched on or activated in the human before the two-cell stage, and probably not before the four-cell stage, even though the embryonic genetic programme is established at the completion of fertilization. Certainly the zygote includes all the genetic material of the egg cytoplasm as part of its own embryonic constitution. Its nucleus contains both maternal and paternal contributions in its complement of 23 pairs of homologous chromosomes, all of which are replicated before the zygote divides mitotically to produce its first two identical daughter cells. This is directed by maternal messenger RNA, derived from the egg. While this must be considered activity of the zygote, it should not be considered activity of the future human individual. The establishment of the new genetic programme at the completion of fertilization is a necessary, but not a sufficient, condition, for the actualization or coming into being of the new human individual at the embryonic stage of existence. The human individual who is ontologically identical with the future adult could hardly be said to exist before the embryonic genome, including the paternal genes, is switched on. If the embryo's own genome is not activated or expressed, or if it is suppressed, no human individual or offspring results.

A human child might carry the genes for haemophilia, but unless they are expressed the child is not affected by the disease. It simply does not exist before it is expressed through the activity of the appropriate gene. Another way of saying this is that a potential haemophiliac victim is not an actual haemophiliac. In an analogous way, though the zygote is an actual individual living being, it could only be a potential human individual if the newly established embryonic genome has not yet begun to be expressed. Genetic determination in the zygote's genotype must not be confused with its subsequent actualization. We are left with the conclusion that despite the zygote's genetic identity with the future adult, despite the fact that it is itself a living ontological individual, it should only be regarded as a potential human individual, not an actual human individual in an ontological sense. Unless the blueprint of the DNA in the zygote's genotype is activated, it is practically a 'dead letter' and could not be considered a true human individual even if it does produce genetically identical progeny up to the two-or four-cell stage before degenerating.

(ii)   *Identical twinning in the zygote*
The sperm and ovum are genetically distinct and living ontological individuals. Their pronuclei mix at syngamy to form a genetically
unique zygote which is itself another distinct living ontological individual.
There is no doubt that the whole human being develops from the zygote,
and that its genetic constitution determines for the most part the developmental process of the embryo to the adult stage. For this reason the zygote
is said to be totipotent, i.e. it is able to develop into a complete human
individual. But does this mean that the zygote is already a human
individual simply because a human being will be derived from it through
developmental processes of differentiation and growth? This argument,
based on the developmental capacity of the zygote, can be seriously
challenged. In this context an egg that is parthenogenetically activated, be
it naturally or artificially, should be regarded the same as one fertilized by
a sperm if it has the same developmental potential.

The same zygote has the natural capacity to become one or more
human beings by virtue of its own inherent active potentiality, when it
cleaves through the process of mitosis into the first two cells or blastomeres. Like the zygote these first two daughter cells are totipotent – each
one can develop into a complete living human individual. Nobody knows
the precise cause or real causes of identical (monozygotic) twinning. It
could possibly be due to an inherited genetic predisposition though there
is no evidence to prove that this is the case. Most probably the cause is
environmental, induced as a result of reduced adhesive qualities in the
substance in contact with the multiplying cells. This factor could itself be
inherited without any need of postulating a genetic predisposition to
twinning in the zygote.

Whatever the cause of monozygotic twinning in the zygote at the two-
cell stage, the fact that it cleaves into two individual blastomeres that may
develop separately as identical twins does not mean the zygote itself is not
a true ontological individual. We know it is a living ontological individual.
But once it divides mitotically into two separate twin daughter blastomeres, it apparently ceases to exist and loses its ontological individuality
to give rise to two new genetically identical, but distinct living ontological
individuals within the zona pellucida. This contains, protects and holds
them together during their early development. The continuity of the same
ontological individual ceases when the zygote forms twins. The zygote is
not the same ontological individual as either one of the eventual twins that
result from its development, notwithstanding its genetic identity continuing throughout all its subsequent cleavages.

But once we assume that the zygote is a human individual because it has the natural active potential to develop into an adult we begin to run into difficulties. The same zygote would also have the natural active potential to develop into two human individuals by the same criteria. We could legitimately ask whether the zygote itself would be one or two human individuals. It would seem absurd to suggest that at the same time it could both be one and more than one human individual, granted that each must be a distinct ontological individual.

It is to be noted, in passing, that this line of reasoning does not only apply to those zygotes that actually do give rise to identical twins. It applies across the board to all zygotes, in so far as they all have the natural active potential to form identical twins that may develop into adults, given suitable conditions. Theoretically this could also be done artificially by the micromanipulation of early human embryos. This means the natural capacity or potential to twin is already present in all zygotes. Twinning only occurs if separate development is induced by some, as yet unknown, causal factor in the environment or within the embryo. The constricting influence of the zona pellucida usually keeps the cleaving cells in close contact and thereby prevents twinning occurring at that stage.

Granted, for the sake of argument, without conceding, that the original parent zygote was an actual human individual, it would be paradoxical, but still necessary, to admit that the original zygote and human individual cease to exist, when, without dying and without a dead cell remaining, it gives asexual origin to identical twin offspring. The two cells resulting from the first cleavage of the zygote would have the same developmental totipotency as the zygote itself. Like the zygote, they would also be human individuals, facing the same fate when they in turn cleaved. The hypothesis of zygotes being persons that cease to exist upon cleaving has little appeal. It would be more realistic to abandon the thesis of the zygote being a human individual in favour of it being the progenitor cell and originating source of all the genetically identical live cells that eventually become one or more human individuals in the course of normal development.

Theoretically there is a possible way out of this dilemma for one who wishes to support fertilization as the starting point for the human individual. Instead of assuming, as I have just done above, that the zygote loses its ontological individuality when it cleaves to form two new distinct identical twins, it could be argued that the original zygote retains its ontological identity when it cleaves and forms only one new individual human being. In this way, both the original zygote and its newly asexually generated single-cell offspring could develop separately to become adult persons in due time. There would appear to be no absurdity or contradiction involved in this. The zygote could be regarded as one human individual that loses a considerable amount of its living matter in the process of giving origin to a new living human individual by mitotic cleavage, without loss of its own ontological individuality. The zygote in this case could be said to produce its own human clone.

This theoretical solution relies on the validity of the analogy of this case with that of a plant giving origin to a new individual plant when a slip is cut off and planted in the soil. We could also recall the example of a human person producing individual live sperm or ova. In these instances there would be one live individual retaining its ontological individuality while it gives origin to another live individual (plant, sperm or ovum). Hence in theory, it would appear that a zygote could retain its individuality and personal identity when cleaving to produce another human individual identical to itself. Put this way, it would appear that, theoretically, identical twinning in itself need not necessarily be incompatible with the zygote being a human individual from the completion of fertilization.

However, human individuals do not resemble plants in this respect. It seems that the analogy used to avoid the dilemma does not apply. The case of an amoeba or a bacterial cell becoming two by fission would be the appropriate analogy to employ in the case of identical twinning in human zygotes. The original parent cell loses its ontological individuality and ceases to exist when two offspring result from the equal sharing of its genetic material. The parent individual actually ceases to exist when the two new ones begin to exist.

It is not enough to consider in the abstract the concept of one individual giving rise to two individuals. It is also necessary to learn from experience how this concretely takes place in each type of living creature. This is required to establish if it is a case of one individual retaining its ontological identity throughout, while it produces its twin, or if it is a case of one individual losing its individuality and separate existence in the process of sharing its genetic material almost equally between two new living identical twin progeny. This latter instance would be the case of binary fission in bacteria, the amoeba and most protozoa. More importantly, I believe the evidence strongly points in the same direction in the case of identical twinning in the human zygote. It is not a human being that loses its ontological individuality but only a single-cell human zygote when monozygotic twinning occurs at this early stage. Inductive rather than deductive reasoning is to be employed to reach a plausible conclusion in this case.

Suppose for a moment that the original zygote, *John*, retained his ontological individuality in the process of producing another genetically identical individual, *Tom*. In the process *John* would be reduced in size by half. This hypothesis would furthermore raise insoluble problems to provide objective and adequate criteria to differentiate between the original *John* and the new individual *Tom* in themselves, quite apart from any difficulties that would be experienced by any eventual observer in trying to do so. Since both twins would be identical in every respect after the division of the zygote, it would be impossible to provide adequate criteria to determine which one was *John*. Both would be identical indiscernibles, except for their separate concrete existences. It would seem to accord more with reason and the facts to accept that the original zygote, be it a person or not, ceases to exist when the two identical twins begin their own separate individual existence. Mitotic cleavage in the zygote should be compared to fission if empirical facts are to guide metaphysical reflection.

It would also be more coherent to hold that whilst admitting the zygote is a living individual being, it could not be a human individual on the simple grounds that, given the right conditions, it had the natural active potentiality to develop into an adult. It could, given the right conditions, equally develop into two adult human individuals. It would have to be both one, and more than one, human individual at the same time. This would be absurd. It is necessary, in practice, to abandon this theoretical attempt to show that the potential for identical twinning in human zygotes is compatible with their personal status based on their natural active capacity to develop into adult persons. The conclusion again would seem to be that a human individual could not be present at the completion of fertilization. The human individual would have to begin at some later stage in the development of the multiplying blastomeres.[21]

(iii)   *The zygote as a human individual in potency*

There is universal agreement that a human child is an actual human individual. This agreement is based on the concept of the human person that we employ. This requires that there be a living multicellular individual of the species *Homo sapiens*. It must be distinct, differentiated and determinate in relation to the organization and integrated articulation of its essential parts, all of whose activities and functions are directed from within for the benefit, well-being, self-development and self-maintenance of the whole individual being. A person must be an individual that has begun to develop its natural capacity to perform acts that are rational, self-conscious, free, and moral. It is not necessary to require complete development of the individual nor the actual exercise of typically personal activities. As stated earlier, we almost unanimously recognize an infant and a fetus several months prior to birth as human beings. This is because we acknowledge there is a real continuing ontological identity between the fetus and the child as the same distinct individual, notwithstanding obvious differences in development. An incompletely developed multi-cellular individual may be a human individual, provided the *same individual* has the natural active potentiality or capacity for truly human development and the exercising, in due time, of typically personal acts of self-reflective knowledge and love.

We need to pursue further the requirements for the continuing onto-logical identity of an individual human being. It is necessary to see if a zygote could be the same living ontological individual as the human adult that develops from it. Undoubtedly the human zygote is a living onto-logical individual with its own characteristic arrangement of its specific, qualitatively heterogeneous, quantitative parts, endowed with activities to serve its self-maintenance and self-development. The same could very well be said, however, of each of its first two identical daughter cells. They also are totipotent. Each would likewise qualify as a distinct ontological individual, notwithstanding the interactions that result from the contacts of their contiguous membranes. The original zygote, as we have already seen, apparently ceases to exist as an ontological individual when it cleaves to give origin to two totipotent cells that are distinct individuals but are nevertheless genetically identical to the parent zygote. This points to a break in the continuity of existence of the zygote as a distinct ontological individual. Two distinct subjects of life appear where there was one, hence the zygote could not be the same ontological individual as its identical daughter cells. It would be even more difficult to hold that the zygote actually is the same ontological individual as the multicellular adult human individual that subsequently develops from it in accord with its genetic instructions. The mere capacity of the zygote to give origin to a fetus, child and adult in itself alone, does not seem to warrant holding that a continuing ontological identity endures from zygote to fetus and to the adult human individual. In other words, the zygote is a human individual in potency, not an actual human individual.

The zygote is already a specifically determined and differentiated ontological individual in itself, but as yet indeterminate and undifferentiated with respect to the individual fetus and child that will develop from it. The individual existence and essential determination of a human zygote is not that of a multicellular fetus or adult human individual. The acorn has the potential to be activated by the warmth and moisture of the soil to become an oak seedling but it is not yet actually an oak seedling. The living zygote's cytoplasm and its vital DNA blueprint for genetically unique development is not yet the one or more multicellular and differentiated human individuals that may be developed from it in due time.

The specific potency of the zygote may be understood by considering what happens to its progeny as cell proliferation and differentiation proceed. We shall return to this issue in the next chapter (see Fig. 5.5). For the present it suffices to note that the first three cleavages produce eight distinct undifferentiated and almost totipotent cells. After this, cell specialization begins during which the ball of cells or morula (= mulberry), first differentiate into two lineages, i.e. trophoblast and the inner cell mass (ICM). Extraembryonic membrane tissues develop from the trophoblast whilst extraembryonic, as well as purely embryonic tissues, develop from the ICM. The zygote has the potential both to produce cells that will form extraembryonic structures that are not strictly constitutive parts of the future definitive embryo proper and fetus and other cells that will only form structures for the definitive embryo proper and fetus. Prior to this differentiation all the cells can give rise to both embryonic and extraembryonic structures. It is this indeterminate state of the zygote both in relation to the differentiation required for the formation of the definitive embryo proper and the number of definitive embryos to be formed that suggests the zygote itself is only potentially a human individual, but not yet an actual human individual.

(iv)   *The life process of the zygote and personhood*

Life is a process; it continues and no longer starts anew. Individuals are the subjects in which the life processes inhere and occur. Individuals begin and cease to live – they begin and cease to be the subjects of the life process. An individual itself is not a process nor can it be reduced to a process. The fact that one live individual develops from another may, or may not, mean they are ontologically identical. A fetus develops to give rise to a baby and is rightly ontologically identified with the baby because it is the same living individual being. It cannot be concluded from this that the fetus, which derives from a zygote, is to be ontologically identified with the zygote unless it can be shown that the zygote is the same living individual being as the fetus. Genetic continuity in life processes does not guarantee continuity of the ontological identity of the individual or individuals involved. In fact, identical twinning shows that it is possible to have continuity of biological life processes with discontinuity of the individual concrete subject of existence. One living individual becomes two with the same genome's life processes continuing unimpeded.

It is not always easy to identify the subject(s) of the developmental life processes. Discrete quantitative criteria and independence of behaviour are useful criteria to apply. Discrete quantities of matter or physical separation indicate distinct individuals in everyday experience of life. Independence of behaviour would tell that a fetus is distinct from the person of the mother or that a virus is distinct from the person of a patient. Sperm and ovum lose their distinct individualities sometime during the long process of fertilization to give origin to a new individual, the zygote. There is no doubt about this even though it is difficult to identify the precise moment in which this distinct new living individual begins. For some it is the moment of penetration of the sperm into the cytoplasm of the egg, for myself syngamy, while for others again it would be the formation of the first mitotic spindle. Our disagreements on exactly when the zygote as a newly formed genetically unique single cell begins does not mean that it does not begin. It is helpful to be aware of these various views concerning the precise stage for the beginning of the zygote.

These same criteria seem to suggest that the zygote loses its ontological individuality when it first cleaves to give origin to two identical daughter blastomeres, quite irrespective of the eventuality of the phenomenon of identical twinning occurring. Two new distinct individuals begin even if they are held in close contact with each other by the zona pellucida for many hours. This view seems to fit the facts better than to hold that a two-celled individual begins at the first cleavage, especially when both cells are totipotent. We are left with the conclusion that the life process of the zygote continues in two new individual subjects after the first cleavage. This means there is no continuity of ontological identity between the zygote and its two daughter cells and consequently between it and the human individual. The zygote could not be the same human individual that is born subsequently.

There are many activities and functions in human individuals that serve obvious purposes. One might think of the respiratory, digestive or circulatory systems. They can be said to be purposive, goal-directed or teleological activities. They continue to serve their purpose so long as the individual is alive, e.g. the digestion of one's food. These activities that promote self-development and self-maintenance are indicators of biological and ontological individuality. They are immanent activities that take place from within for the benefit of the living individual as a whole.

The human reproductive process is likewise purposive and goal directed. Nobody would deny that its purpose is to give birth to a healthy baby. All the goal-directed activities of the reproductive process, however, do not belong to one ontological individual. Fetal and maternal activities and responses are wondrously co-ordinated for the benefit of the fetus without any suggestion that these activities belong only to one individual. Mitosis is a purposive process directed from within the zygote. This does not mean that it results in a two-celled individual rather than two individual cells. Purposefulness of living activities alone cannot determine if they are the activities of one individual or interactions between more than one individual. Other criteria, as we have seen, are needed to settle this issue. The reproductive purpose of mitosis alone cannot determine that the first cleavage of the zygote leaves a two-celled ontological individual rather than two cells, each of which is a living ontological individual. The purposefulness of mitosis in the zygote does not resolve the issue in favour of continuity of ontological individuality of the zygote from fertilization onwards. The previous conclusion stands: the zygote does not seem to be the same living individual as the one or more human individuals that are derived from it.

(v)   *Biological human nature and ontological human individuation*

There is no doubt that the product of the fertilization of human gametes is a human zygote, a human embryo, biologically belonging to the human species. It is not feline or canine. Speaking genetically and biologically we may say its nature is human. The cells of an adult human have the same genetic constitution or nature as that of the original zygote from which they are derived. Hybrids apart, the biological nature of each individual mammal, man included, is determined at the completion of fertilization when the zygote is actually constituted. In this biological sense we may say that the human zygote belongs to the species *Homo sapiens*, that it is a human type of living being or simply that it is a *human* being as distinct from a being of any other species. It is possible to use the expression *human being* in a purely biological sense without employing it to mean also a person in either its ordinary or philosophical sense. This seems to have been the meaning of the evidence given by Professor Lejeune, an outstanding French geneticist, to the Australian *Senate Select Committee on the Human Embryo Experimentation Bill 1985*:

...it is bewildering to hear now in our time, with all that demonstration and experimental evidence that we have in our species that man begins at fecundation, speculation – not about the facts, because the facts are clear – but about the interpretation of the facts, and some people say a human embryo has not yet humanised. I must say very simply, as a geneticist, I have never heard any specialist in husbandry of animals thinking about the 'cattlisation' of cattle. They know that the embryo of a cow would be a calf... From all the genetic laws that we have tried to summarise, we are entirely convinced that every embryo is, by itself, a human being.[22]

Professor Lejeune emphasized the continuity of the same human nature from the embryo to death further on in his evidence:

So I would say that what is constant is its nature, and I would say that an embryo has fully the human nature just as much as the foetus has a full human nature and as much as the school boy and a grown up or an old man. That is a human nature that is entirely constant from fecundation to normal death.[23]

One could not be blamed for thinking that Professor Lejeune held that an individual human being existed from the completion of the process of fertilization if he maintains that a complete human nature begins to be present from that time onwards. It is interesting to read his evidence to an American Senate Sub-committee on the Separation of Powers in April 1981 on human individuation, understood genetically:

As it was ... demonstrated by Market [*sic*] and Peter [*sic*], a chimeric mouse can derive from two or even three embryos, but no more. The maximum number of cells cooperating to the elaboration of an individual is three. In full accordance with this empirical demonstration, which was available to science last year, the fertilized egg normally cleaves itself into two cells, one of them dividing again, thus forming the surprising odd number of three cells, encapsulated inside their protective bag, the zona pellucida. To the best of our actual knowledge, the prerequisite for individuation – that is, a stage containing three fundamental cells – is the next step following conception, minutes after it.[24]

Professor Lejeune is here effectively asserting that the individual human being or person could not begin before the three-cell stage, even though a biologically human nature begins once fertilization is completed with the formation of the unicellular zygote. His grounds for this assertion rest on the fact that a chimaeric mouse can be formed from cells derived from no more than three different mouse embryos. It is difficult to see any connection or relevance of the facts with this assertion of Lejeune. But he is prepared to locate individuation at some stage after fertilization.

On closer examination of the work of Markert and Petters it appears that Lejeune has misunderstood the results of their research. They were not referring to the first three cells of the embryo at all. In a hexaparental mouse blastocyst of 64 cells, from 10 to 15 cells make up the inner cell mass (ICM) and of *these only three* have been found to contribute to the resultant live chimaeric mouse that showed signs of three different cell lines in its genetic constitution. They stated their conclusion quite clearly:

> Our data and that of others suggest that three cells and only three cells in the ICM of the blastocyst are the sole source of the cells making up the adult. The vast majority of cells in the blastocyst never contribute to the tissues of the adult.[25]

If Lejeune had interpreted their research correctly, he would probably have concluded that individuation did not occur in the human blastocyst before the inner cell mass had formed about five days after fertilization instead of after about 36 hours when the third cell would have appeared.

Our conclusion is that human nature, understood in a genetic or biological sense, begins at the completion of fertilization so that only a human being could normally develop from a human zygote. Monozygotic twins that result from a single human zygote are also genetically identical. This means that both the human genetic constitution or nature as well as the genetic identity of the one or more human individuals that may develop are already determined at the zygote stage. What is not determined is the number of human individuals that will be the subjects or bearers of that genetically determined human nature present in the zygote produced from human gametes. In short, the zygote is certainly a biologically human cell, but apparently not yet a human individual in an ontological sense. The conclusion seems quite clear: the human zygote, though possessed of a biological human nature, could not be an actual human individual but only a human progenitor cell with the natural active potency to develop only into one or more human individuals but not a member of another species. This is so because ontological human individuation is a prior condition for the formation of a person, i.e. a distinct on-going ontological individual with a biological human nature.

(vi)   *Philosophical theories and biological facts*

We have seen how empirical methods of investigation fail to notice philosophically significant discontinuity of existence in the cleaving zygote. In fact the scientists quoted above (see pp. 115–16) spoke about the beginning of human development, or the human individual or human being in a biological sense of the terms. The *uniqueness* referred to was genetic. They certainly were not trying to refer to a human individual in any ontological sense as a pre-requisite for human personhood. It would be quite misleading to conclude from their empirical definitions that a human individual in an ontological sense or as a person begins at fertilization. Keith Moore suggests some ambiguity when he explains the meaning of the term *embryo*, as distinct from zygote referred to above (p. 115) as follows.

> This term refers to the developing human during the early stages of development. The term is usually not used until the second week, after the embryonic disc forms.[26]

Dorland's Illustrated Medical Dictionary is far more scientific when it defines *zygote* as 'the cell after synapsis at the completion of fertilization until first cleavage'.[27] Likewise a scientifically accurate definition is given for embryo: 'In man, the developing organism is an embryo from about two weeks after fertilization to the end of seventh or eighth week.'[28]

By the same token philosophy as such will not be able to answer empirical or factual questions. We have to examine the evidence to see how a new human individual arises and apply the philosophical principles correctly to explain the facts. Understood in this way, Aristotelian–Thomistic philosophical principles in theory could equally account for the origin of the human person either at fertilization, or after it. It all depends on the relevant scientific biological evidence and its interpretation. As we have seen, philosophers do use the same scientific biological facts to defend different philosophical positions.

These same philosophical principles are also quite adequate to account for the origin and constitution of many individuals in the same species. The principles of *actuality* and *potentiality*, *matter* and *form*, coupled with bodies' quantitative requirements, are perfectly adequate to explain everything and solve the problems that arise. Once we are sure we have the beginning of a human individual, it is quite understandable to speak of a person with potential to indicate that this human being is still in the developmental stages. As needed, allowance is to be made for many degrees of potency – from remote to proximate.

I do also think, however, that some who openly profess Aristotelian–Thomistic philosophical principles, surreptitiously, albeit unwittingly, are influenced by philosophical dualism when it comes to establishing the beginning of the human person in a zygote. I suspect that a Platonic or Cartesian dualistic interpretation of the body–mind relationship, especially before the discovery of the genetic make-up of the zygote, could also have supported the conviction that a human person is present from the completion of fertilization. There is some appeal in the thought that the spiritual soul, created with its own autonomous ontological identity, dualistically unites with the zygote to form a person that gradually differentiates under its guiding and organizing influence. Perhaps they are also misled by the singular grammatical form of the term *embryo* into believing that it must refer to an on-going natural entity (ontological individual) and consequently a person from fertilization onwards. It is easy to be mesmerized by the grammatical form of language itself.

These appealing thoughts should not dispense philosophers from carefully examining the biological facts before proposing philosophical solutions to the problem of the beginning of the human individual. The trouble with the traditional view is that it uncritically assumes that the human person is present from fertilization, and then provides a possible explanation for its fully human development. The right way is surely to make philosophical theories fit the facts rather than ignore or select the facts to suit a preferred philosophical theory. One should not postulate the presence of a spiritual soul, informing or animating a body, before one is assured of the actual presence of an ontological individual that is a person by reason of its complete human nature.

The dual principles of spiritual soul (form) and matter, or more simply mind and body, are introduced to explain adequately the unity and functioning of the human person, understood as a primitive and underived datum of our experience. They do not pre-exist the human person, as though they *come together* to form the human being. They begin to exist as constitutive co-principles of a person only when the ontological individual human being is actually present. It is difficult to see how this could be so before the actual formation of a truly multicellular individual living body. Its specific heterogeneous quantitative parts would be needed for the activities required for orderly self-development, self-maintenance, self-differentiation and growth. It would also be necessary that its life-cycle proceed within the same continuing ontological individual. This is so if we are to be true to the facts of experience and our basic conceptual framework for thinking about human persons. It is extremely difficult to maintain that the human individual begins at fertilization itself. The evidence seems to be insufficient to warrant drawing any conclusions beyond that of the zygote being one or more human individuals, in potency.

5

Implantation and the beginning of the human individual

It is now necessary to examine the stages of embryonic development after fertilization to see when the human individual begins. This will be done by way of exclusion by attempting to establish the last stage, or time, prior to which it would appear impossible, or at least implausible, for a human individual to be present in an ontological sense. In the following pages I shall first consider why it would seem that the individual human person could not be present during the early cleavage stage before the formation of the morula. In this section I will further discuss the implications of identical twinning for the beginning of the human individual, even though identical twinning can occur beyond this stage right up until implantation is almost completed. Arguments will then be presented that favour delaying hominization, or the formation of the human individual, beyond compaction and the morula stage. Next I will consider the relevance of naturally occurring short-lived parthenogenetic development that probably does occasionally occur in the human species. Finally, I shall examine evidence that suggests that the human individual could not actually exist before the formation of the blastocyst and its successful implantation in the womb about 13 days after fertilization.

1 The human individual not present during the early cleavage stage
(i) *Possibility of identical twinning during the early cleavage stage*

It is important to bear in mind that the development of eutherian mammalian embryos differs quite significantly from that of amphibians. Of crucial importance for the former is the prior formation of extra-embryonic tissues and membranes (e.g. placenta), whereas the latter have no such need. The mammalian zygote cleaves in two, dividing the cytoplasm in more or less equal parts, but not along any predetermined axis.

Unlike the amphibian, the human zygote is not regionally determined in relation to its cytoplasmic contents. This is shown by the capacity of randomly divided early blastomeres to produce viable monozygotic twins or even quadruplets up to the eight-cell stage. If anything, initial regional distinctions result from responses to environmental cues.[1] The early blastomeres tend to cleave along an axis that will yield rounded cells.

The first cleavage produces two identical cells of about equal size, each with 46 chromosomes. Each cell is an individual living being that is distinct and totipotent. Each is able to give rise to an adult human being. Whatever potential is possessed by the original fertilized egg is also possessed by each of its daughter cells. The existence of monozygotic or identical twins from the two-cell stage suggests in a convincing way, as we have already seen, that the fertilized ovum is far from being actually organized into a single continuing ontological human individual. When this occurs at the two-cell stage, each cell becomes a separate blastocyst, each twin having its own amnion, chorion and placenta, i.e. dichorial twins.

It is this sort of information about the number of extraembryonic membranes in relation to the fetus that enables the approximate timing of the event of identical twinning to be determined. According to R. G. Edwards, 32% of identical twins are dichorial and begin at the two-blastomere stage, while 68% are monochorial and begin approximately between three–eight days after fertilization.[2] These latter probably are caused by a splitting of the loosely adhesive cells of the inner cell mass (ICM) within the blastocyst by chance, or possibly during their 'hatching out' of the zona pellucida if it happens to be still hard or resistant. (How many cooks have accidentally broken the yolk when shelling eggs before frying them!) Monoamniotic twins are very rare and occur between eight and 12 days after fertilization, or even later in the case of conjoined twins that fail to separate completely.[3] The actual incidence of identical twinning varies slightly from country to country, but the average is about three–four per 1000 births.[4] The sharing of membranes and common placenta by monochorial and monoamniotic identical twins would seem to argue against considering them as constitutive organs of each embryo or developing fetus, even though they are needed for support and survival (see Fig. 5.1). This is a sign that the shared organ may be functionally vital for both without being an exclusive part of either. The functioning of an artificial kidney is vital, but not a part of the human individual.

It has been found that identical twinning occurs in embryos where first cell specification may be detected by experimental methods up to the 32-

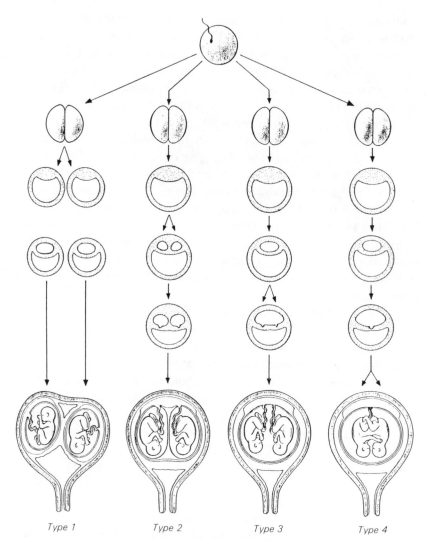

Type 1   Type 2   Type 3   Type 4

Fig. 5.1. Arrangement of the fetal membranes in different types of monozygotic twin pregnancies. *Type 1:* separate membranes = dichorionic twins.
Separation of the zygote occurred at the two-blastomere stage (1–3 days
after fertilization). *Type 2:* the most frequent: one placenta, separate
amnions = monochorionic diamniotic twins. Separation of the zygote occurred
at the inner cell mass – early blastocyst stage (3–8 days) *Type 3:* completely
common membranes = monoamniotic twins. Separation at the embryonic disc
stage (8–12 days). *Type 4:* completely common membranes and yolk sac, and
only partial separation of embryos, which can take place at any of several later
stages = Siamese or conjoined twins. Type 1 occurs also in dizygotic twins, but
Types 2, 3 and 4 can only involve monozygotic twins. (Partly redrawn from

cell stage or more. This holds for mammals, amphibians and sea urchins. Identical twinning does not occur where cell specification can already be detected in embryos with two to eight cells, e.g. the ascidian, annelid, mollusc or the ctenophore. The possibility of twinning is obviously related to a sufficiently large number of cells being still in a relatively unspecified or undifferentiated state.[5] Identical twinning can only take place where the cells or cluster of cells, when divided, possess a regulatory potential that is totipotential by reason of the number and uncommitted state of the cells.

These facts show that not only the zygote but also the developing cluster of cells for many days afterwards has the capacity to separate and thereby allow independent development to proceed and form more than one human being. Recent research has shown that there is a slight genetic predisposition to monozygotic twinning. It was found that the incidence of monozygotic twinning among the maternal relatives of identical twins is significantly higher than the incidence found in the general population. This would indicate that some propensity to monozygotic twinning could be inherited through the maternal line.[6] This alone, however, is unable to account for the majority of cases of monozygotic twinning. As suggested earlier, internal or external chance factors seem to account for most instances of identical twinning. A factor could be inherited that facilitates identical twinning (e.g. predisposition to form weak glue-like desmosomes that bind cells together) without implying that identical twinning was genetically predetermined.

The evidence shows that a single-cell human zygote and a cluster of cells may cleave to give origin to twins that develop separately to become adult human individuals. There are no valid reasons or evidence to suggest that a human individual cleaves or divides by mitosis or fission to give origin to twin persons. Indeed, as we have already seen, the contrary is the case. If the natural active potentiality of the zygote and cluster of cells to develop into an adult person were enough to constitute an actual person, we would have to claim that the zygote and cluster of cells at the same time, was both one person and more than one person. We cannot accept this at all, so it would be reasonable to deny that the zygote and cluster of cells are persons on the simple grounds of their potentiality or inherent capacity to

---

Caption for fig. 5.1 (*cont.*)

H. Tuchmann-Duplessis, G. David and P. Haegel. *Illustrated Human Embryology*, vol. 1. Springer-Verlag, New York; Chapman and Hall, London; Masson et Cie, Paris (1971).) (From C. R. Austin and R. V. Short, *Embryonic and Fetal Development, Reproduction in Mammals* Bk 2, Cambridge: C.U.P., 1982.)

develop into one or more than one adult person. Loss of ontological individuality by the zygote or cluster of cells when they cleave is a crucial consideration in this case.

One could suppose, as we have already done for the zygote, that the cluster of cells really was a multicellular individual embryo – a person, say *Susan*. When twinning occurs, *Susan*, as one whole living individual would asexually give origin to her twin sister. There would be the same difficulties that we experienced in the case of the zygote to establish which embryo was really *Susan*. This, in its turn, would lead to the suggestion that *Susan*, as in the case of the zygote, would cease to exist in giving origin to her identical twin offspring, *Margaret* and *Sally*. In this case these would be the grandchildren of their unsuspecting mother and father! This exercise gets us no further than when we were discussing the same issue in the case of zygotes. A multicellular embryo that was an ontological individual capable of twinning would lose its ontological individuality in the process. In other words, there could not be the same human individual present before and after the twinning process, notwithstanding the continuing genetic identity present in each twin.

Rather than accept that a human individual ceased to exist in the twinning process, it would be more plausible to argue that an ontological human individual had not yet begun to exist. An individual that was capable of becoming one or more persons could only be a potential person, not a distinct actual person as we have argued already in the case of the zygote. The same would apply for a cluster of individual cells with the same capacity. They would have the potential to become persons – twins, triplets or even quadruplets upon dividing, but would not yet be an actual person. There is no evidence to suggest an individual person ever ceases to exist when twinning occurs.

It would appear possible that at least in some cases identical twins could originate as a result of an inherited genetic factor present in the genes of the DNA in the zygote. This factor could be triggered any time after the first mitotic cleavage during the following 10–12 days. In these hypothetical cases the monozygotic twinning would be predetermined from the very beginning to occur at a particular stage of development of the embryo. In this case, even the traditionalist would probably agree that the individual person could not be actually individuated and constituted until the mysterious factor was activated and twinning did occur. This hypothesis certainly makes it easier to think that if hominization, or the actual beginning of human personhood, could be delayed in some cases during embryonic development, it could be delayed in all cases. These reflections make the possibility of the delayed origin of distinct individual persons sound perfectly feasible. In saying this, I do not intend this hypothesis alone to be taken as a valid argument in favour of delayed hominization for embryos that are not programmed to twin. Further evidence would need to be found and analysed critically before suggesting when all human individuals might actually begin during embryonic development.

(ii)   *Lack of unity in the early human embryo*

There is very little evidence of intrinsic unity, or of the presence of a single individual organism, in the first cleavages of the cells in the human embryo (see Fig. 5.2). Their membranes merely touch within the zona pellucida. They remain totipotential up to the four-cell stage but possibly not much further.[7] Mohr and Trounson report that primitive junctional complexes have been seen as early as the eight-cell stage, although the characteristic tight junctions are not formed until the morula stage of about 32 cells.[8] They would be referring initially to desmosomes, or glue-like junctions, that hold the cells loosely together. The tight junctions act as permeable seals. Hence, it appears that at least up to the eight-cell stage in the human embryo there are eight distinct individuals rather than one multicellular individual.[9] It is the zona pellucida that gives the appearance of a single organism or unity by holding the eight distinct individual cells together. It prevents them from coming apart and sticking to the walls of the fallopian tube and protects them during their journey to the womb. The embryo enters the womb from the two–three day stage when it has between 8 and 16 cells.[10]

The cytoplasm of the egg contains nutrients to sustain the metabolic activities of the living human zygote and the cells that it produces. Each of these contains its own share of cytoplasmic nutrients on a diminishing scale as the number of mitotic divisions increases and the cells become progressively smaller. Some nutrients are also taken in from the environment. Glycoproteins and glycogens are absorbed by diffusion from the fluids in the oviduct and uterus. At this stage nutrients are used to supply the energy needs for cell division, not for growth, which occurs only after the blastocyst stage and implantation. By this time, nutrients are supplied from the maternal blood stream by way of the syncytiotrophoblastic lacunae at first, and finally through the placenta. Once implantation is completed the embryo proper grows rapidly.[11] Prior to implantation, and more obviously when there are no more than eight blastomeres, each cell takes in its own nutrients, thereby showing autonomy in a vitally significant way. This would indicate that each blastomere at least up to the

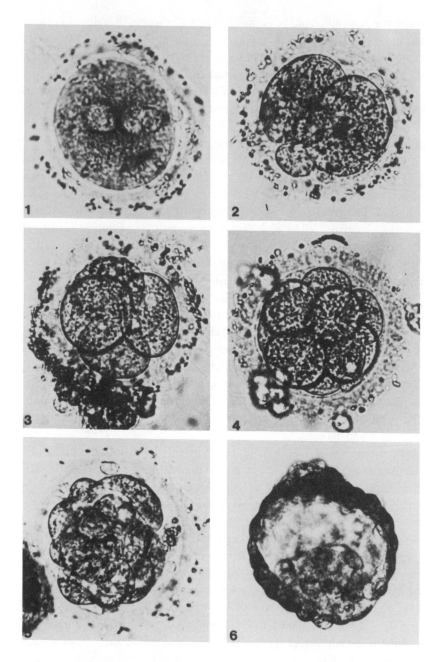

Fig. 5.2. **Preimplantation human embryos**. Photograph key: 1. A 1-cell human embryo 12 hours after fertilization; 2. A 2-cell human embryo 30 hours; 3. A 4-cell human embryo 40 hours; 4. An 8-cell human embryo 55 hours;

eight-cell stage was a distinct ontological living individual, even if the life span of each blastomere consisted of less than 24 hours.

We are left with the conclusion that the early human embryo is really a cluster of distinct individual cells, each one of which is a centrally organized living individual or ontological entity in simple contact with the others enclosed in the protective zona pellucida. It would be difficult to justify attributing the natural unity proper to a single ontological individual to the cluster of cells as a whole. We should not confuse the unity of the future human individual with the actual four–eight undifferentiated homogeneous cells that are oriented to become that same human individual through a continuous process of development. We should resist the conceptual and linguistic temptation to attribute an unwarranted ontological unity to an actual multiplicity of developing human blastomeres.

(iii)   *Animal experiments suggest absence of unity and actual determination for the ontological human individual in the early embryo*

Further evidence that the embryo during the early cleavage stage has not yet become a distinct ontological human individual can be found in some interesting experiments with animal embryos. The phenomenon of monozygotic twinning suggests that the early blastomeres of sheep and mouse embryos could easily be disaggregated and be variously combined by techniques of micromanipulation.[12] This enables blastomeres from different embryos to be aggregated until blastulation occurs in evacuated zonae, sealed with agar in a cylinder. This is then placed within the temporary womb of a pseudo-pregnant sheep or mouse, before the blastocysts are transferred to a permanent host womb. Chimaeric mice and sheep have been produced by these techniques, clearly showing a mixture of the various colours or other traits of their original parent blastomeres or embryos. Embryos can be both disaggregated and/or

---

Caption for fig. 5.2 (*cont.*)

5. A morula stage human embryo 100 hours; 6. A blastocyst stage human embryo 140 hours after fertilization. All these embryos have been photographed alive, in sterile culture media, using a non-invasive technique. (Reproduced with permission from *The Journal of Reproduction and Fertility*, and the authors, Trounson, A. O., Mohr, L., Wood, C. and Leeton, J. F., with the permission of Dr A. Trounson.)

joined together without significant loss of developmental potential to survive and be born alive.

Much can be learnt about the developmental capacity of human embryos by studying how blastomeres of some animals regulate their development subsequent to the micromanipulation of these cells at the cleavage stage. It has been found that isolated cells from the two-cell stage develop more successfully than those from the four-cell stage and the eight-cell stage respectively. This is most likely due to the fact that only the earlier and larger blastomeres could produce enough cells for blastulation to succeed at the predetermined species-specific time. A minimum complement of cell mass would be required for each species. Sheep embryos blastulate at about the 64-cell stage whereas mouse embryos do so at about the 32-cell stage. This would explain why blastomeres isolated at the two-, four- and eight-cell stage in the sheep have a greater probability of producing live young than in the mouse.

The developmental capacity of pairs of blastomeres from the *same* or *different* embryos at various stages is constant. Aggregates of two cells from different embryos at the two-cell stage or two halves from different embryos at the four-cell or eight-cell stage all demonstrate equal developmental capacity since the overall cell mass or number has not been reduced. It is very difficult to succeed in disaggregating 16-cell embryos and recombining them without fatal damage since by that stage desmosomes, and possibly tight junctions, have already been formed to bind the cells together. Willadsen and Fehilly, however, have shown that lambs can be produced with various success rates from half- and quarter- sheep embryos irrespective of when the reduction in cell number is made, up to and including the eight-cell stage.[13] Half-embryos were at least 70% successful and quarter-embryos were 50% successful. Only 10% of eighth-embryos produced a lamb. Chimaeric quarter-embryos composed of one blastomere from two different eight-cell parent embryos were as viable as non-chimaeric quarter-embryos. Quarter-embryos usually produced non-chimaeric lambs, whereas embryos aggregated from half-embryos derived from two-cell embryos usually were chimaeric. It would appear that the two eighth-blastomeres that made the quarter-embryo had each an equal opportunity of giving rise to the whole ICM from which the future non-chimaeric lamb would eventually develop. The two half-embryos, when combined, would each normally contribute progeny to the ICM and so produce a chimaeric lamb. They also showed that a three-eighth chimaeric embryo, produced by combining a single blastomere from an eight-cell embryo with one from a four-cell embryo, tends to produce a non-chimaeric lamb corresponding to the lineage of the blastomere taken from the eight-cell embryo.

All these techniques enable biochemically labelled cells to be traced right through the development of the fetus to produce 'fate maps' of the progeny of various cell lines (see Fig. 5.5). In this way the various tissues and stages of differentiation can be seen to originate from different parts of the developing embryo, and so reveal its developmental history. Not always do both parent embryo cell lines appear: they are often non-chimaeric, particularly if two blastomeres from different eight-cell embryos are combined. In such cases the progeny of one cell contributes exclusively to the extraembryonic membranes and tissues, while the other's progeny provides the cells for the ICM from which the embryo proper and eventual fetus develops. All this is possible because the blastomeres are combined before the embryos have developed their own immune system. As we shall see, various types of combinations and/or twinning are possible until implantation is completed.

The results of these two researchers in the United Kingdom show that whereas two sheep blastomeres of the same stage of development, when combined, have an equal chance to form the ICM from which the future lamb is developed, this is not the case when blastomeres of different stages of development combine. In short, the more developed blastomere from an eight-cell embryo has less regulatory developmental potential with respect to the less advanced blastomere from the four-cell embryo. The more advanced and smaller blastomere becomes surrounded by the progeny of the less advanced and larger blastomere. Similar results are obtained in experiments with blastomeres from mouse embryos, though less flexibility is shown in their regulatory and developmental potential. No doubt, this is due to the fact that only 32 cells are usually required for mouse embryos to successfully blastulate instead of 64 in the case of sheep. This means the developmental potential of isolated blastomeres is actualized earlier in the mouse than in the sheep, thereby restricting their regulatory capacity at a less advanced stage compared to sheep. Half-mouse embryos produced at the eight-cell stage (i.e. four cells) are viable, whereas quarter (i.e. two cells) and eighth (i.e. one cell) embryos are usually not viable. In this latter case there are insufficient cells to support further development, especially when the set time for blastulation arrives with too few cells being allocated to the ICM.

Various sized chimaeric blastocysts have been constructed by aggregating up to eight times the normal number of blastomeres from the two- to eight-cell stage (see Table 5.1). Frequently the offspring born are also

Table 5.1. *The development of composite sheep embryos produced by aggregation of various numbers of blastomeres from two or more parent embryos at the 2- to 8-cell stage*

| | Composition of embryos | | | | | | | | |
	$\frac{1}{8} + \frac{1}{8}$	$\frac{1}{8} + \frac{1}{4} + \frac{1}{4}$	$4 \times \frac{1}{8}$	$\frac{1}{2} + \frac{1}{2}$	$8 \times \frac{1}{8}$	$8 \times \frac{2}{8}$	$4 \times \frac{8}{8}$	$8 \times \frac{8}{8}$	Total
No. transferred to temporary recipients	21	32	13	5	4	9	19	2	105
No. recovered from temporary recipients	18	28	13	5	4	9	17	2	96
No. of well-integrated blastocysts	16	15	11	5	4	8	12	2	73
No. transferred to definitive recipients	10	15	11	5	4	8	15	2	70
No. of full term lambs	5	10	9	3	4	6	13	2	52
No. blood typed	3	10	9	3	4	6	13	0	48
No. of chimaeras (overt and/or blood)	0	5	6	3	4	6	12	–	36

Notes: $\frac{1}{8}$ denotes one blastomere from an 8-cell embryo; $\frac{1}{4}$ denotes a 4-cell embryo; $\frac{1}{2}$ denotes one blastomere from a 2-cell embryo; $4 \times \frac{1}{8}$ denotes four blastomeres each from a different 8-cell embryo; $\frac{2}{8}$ denotes two blastomeres from a single 8-cell embryo; $8 \times \frac{2}{8}$ denotes eight pairs of blastomeres from eight different 8-cell embryos. (From C. B. Fehilly and S. M. Willadsen, 'Embryo manipulation in farm animals', *Oxford Reviews of Reproductive Biology*, ed. J. R. Clarke, Vol. 8, 1986. Courtesy of the Clarendon Press.)

chimaeric. The largest number of parent embryos which have been proven to be represented in the sheep and the mouse is three. This has been shown by the use of genetic markers or by testing the bloodtypes. It is not certain if three is the absolute maximum, or if that is the most that can be proven with present techniques of embryo manipulation, genetic marking and bloodtyping.[14] When fewer than the normal number of cells for a particular stage are aggregated, the likelihood of non-chimaeric offspring increases since the embryo proper would in all probability develop from only one parent embryo cell line.

It has been found that when non-chimaeric offspring are derived from chimaeric 'quarter-blastocysts' aggregated from two eight-cell sheep embryos ($\frac{1}{8}$A + $\frac{1}{8}$B) they are only immunologically tolerant towards each other provided they were derived from the same parent embryo. This is an interesting discovery in view of the fact that in all such cases the extraembryonic tissues must have been chimaeric, i.e. with the cell lines of both A and B represented in the placenta.[15] Undoubtedly, such an experiment could technically, but not ethically, be done with human embryos. It does suggest that the placenta, though vitally important for the survival of the fetus, is not an organ that strictly constitutes a live part of the embryo proper and fetus itself.

Similar results can be obtained from interspecies chimaerism.[16] It is known that neither the sheep nor the goat will become pregnant as a result of the transfer of an embryo from the opposite species to a recipient female. However, chimaeric sheep–goat half-blastocysts produced by combining one blastomere each from four-cell sheep and goat embryos were able to produce live young after transfer to recipient sheep and goat females. Of the seven offspring born, three were overt sheep–goat chimaeras. A live goat kid was born to a sheep after the transfer of a chimaeric blastocyst developed from two blastomeres from an eight-cell goat embryo and one from a four-cell sheep embryo. This demonstrated that the trophoblast and placental tissues developed from the sheep line, while the goat offspring developed entirely from the cell progeny derived from the goat parent embryo.

An overtly chimaeric ram lamb has been produced by aggregating a blastomere from a four-cell sheep embryo with one from an eight-cell sheep × goat hybrid embryo ($\frac{1}{4}$S + $\frac{1}{8}$H). It is rare to achieve success in introducing the hybrid line into the sheep. On most occasions such experimental micromanipulation of sheep × goat hybrid embryo blastomeres with those of sheep have produced lambs with pure sheep bloodtypes. This is probably because the sheep × goat hybrid embryos develop more slowly than sheep embryos, resulting in the cell progeny of the hybrid blastomeres being allocated for the most part to the trophectoderm at blastulation, while the derivatives of the sheep blastomeres displaced them from contributing to the formation of the embryo proper and fetus from within the ICM.[17]

Though these experimental manipulations have not been performed on human embryos, they do shed some light on the character of the developmental and regulatory potential of the human embryo as well. This is so because of the acknowledged similarity existing in the early stages of embryonic development of all eutherian mammals. The mouse and sheep embryo in particular very closely resemble, but are not identical to, the human embryo in its early developmental stages.[18] This enables much to be learnt about human embryos from experiments with early mouse and sheep embryos, morulae and blastocysts, both before and after the implantation stage.[19]

The importance of these experiments for our purpose derives from the fact that at least up to the four-cell stage of the human embryo its developmental and regulatory potential is similar in many respects to that of the sheep and mouse embryo. This means, furthermore, that each of the first four blastomeres of the human embryo, when combined with a single cell from a different two-cell embryo, could theoretically produce a non-chimaeric fetus and child in due time from a chimaeric blastocyst. This implies that four genetically identical quadruplets could be obtained from one human zygote since only the progeny of the more advanced cell in each case would contribute to the ICM and the embryo proper. The progeny of the less advanced cells would contribute only to the extra-embryonic membranes and tissues. This means the placenta would be genetically different from the fetus. I am not suggesting the ethical feasibility of such manipulations of the human embryo. I am merely suggesting this possibility itself provides little support for the view that an on-going distinct ontological human individual actually begins at the zygote stage or by the four-cell stage.

These experiments with chimaeric embryos show that the chimaeric offspring could not begin before the aggregation of the relevant blasto-meres at the four- and eight-cell stage of development. The genetic dissimilarity of various parts of the offspring is a strong argument against the chimaeric offspring beginning as an ontological individual before the aggregation of the cells from which it is derived. To argue that the original sheep and goat zygotes were already actual individual sheep and goats prior to the aggregation of the chimaeric embryos lacks a sense of realism and appears to be a desperate attempt to prop up the assumption that the zygote is already an on-going ontological individual of the species concerned, be it sheep, goat or human. It would be necessary in this hypothesis to maintain either that both the original individuals ceased to be when the chimaera was formed or that only one survived, incorporating features of the other in its genetic constitution. All things considered, the evidence seems to indicate that non-chimaeric ontological individuals of any eutherian mammalian species (including the human) could not begin to exist before the eight-cell stage, even if the genetic identity were established at the zygote stage for all.

These experiments, especially those with chimaeric embryos, suggest that the developmental potential of fertilized eutherian mammalian eggs and their undifferentiated daughter cells after the first three cleavages is far too indeterminate and unrestricted for a single cell or each cluster of the first eight cells to be considered an actual on-going ontological individual of any species. Furthermore, it would be very difficult, in the light of all the facts, to believe that a cluster of cells is a living individual that retains the same ontological individuality and identity throughout all subsequent stages of development and growth. There is good reason to apply these conclusions to the human zygote and the early preimplanted human embryo. This is so because the fetus is finally derived from some cells that make up the ICM. How could the fetus actually exist if the ICM did not yet exist? Clearly, up to the four-cell stage we could only speak of a potential human individual present in the four cells, each of which is a distinct ontological individual. This fits the facts, whereas to view the eight-cell embryo as one ontological individual, with parts that are potential individuals, seems to conflict with the scientific evidence at hand. If the human embryo could not yet be an individual, but only a cluster of cells, it certainly could not be a human being.

Certainly once cells are disaggregated by micromanipulations, be it at the four- or eight-cell stage, they are undoubtedly separate ontological individuals, at least until they are combined to form new individuals. It is a fact that three or four cells from one sheep embryo can be combined with three or four cells from another sheep embryo to form three or four new chimaeric embryos that produce three or four lambs, chimaeric or non-chimaeric. There should be no particular difficulty in believing that three or four distinct individual cells in the same sheep embryo could combine to form an individual embryo, fetus and live lamb. The same could be said for other combinations. If several cells from *different* sheep or mouse embryos can combine to produce a single lamb or mouse, could it not very well be that several cells derived from the *same* fertilized ovum could likewise form a single sheep or mouse embryo and fetus in the natural situation?

I think we can apply this same line of reasoning to the cells in the human embryo. Many cells that are distinct individuals eventually interact, differentiate, develop and naturally form a single individual embryo, fetus and baby at birth in the normal situation. I think this explanation fits the facts better than to assume there is one and the same individual human being developing from the fertilized-egg stage all the way through to birth. The zona pellucida is a temporary external protector that helps the distinct cells developing from the zygote to form junctions, before they eventually differentiate to form a distinct embryonic human being in a natural process. In this way Nature prevents the dispersal of the cells and favours the formation of one human individual. By way of exception, due to accidental causes, identical twins may be formed instead, or the early embryos may fail to implant in the uterus.

Finally, these researchers merely confirmed the results of Chris Graham and his colleagues at Oxford. They showed that the progeny of the first cell to divide at the two-cell stage of the mouse embryo contributed more cells to the inner cell mass than to the outer cells of the trophectoderm.[20] Presumably, the same would apply to the human embryo in the normal situation, so that the first advanced human blastomere would have a greater determining influence on the subsequent development of the human embryo. While this is a further argument against the fertilized ovum being an actual human person, I do not at all suggest this in itself is a convincing argument for considering the three-cell human embryo to be sufficiently determined and individuated to constitute an individual human being. The actualization of a distinct ontological human individual, rather than the potency for its realization in a unique embryonic genome, is the hallmark of a true human individual.

2   The human individual not present during the morula stage

Up to the eight-cell stage the blastomeres are all distinct, toti-potential, undifferentiated homogeneous cells with the same state of specification. From this stage onwards some differences begin to appear. They can no longer continue to divide in such a way as to produce rounded blastomeres due to the lack of inter-blastomeric space within the constricting confines of the zona pellucida. Hence a process of compaction occurs between the 8- and 16-cell stage, whereby the cells and/or cell surfaces exposed to the outside become less adhesive and covered with microvilli, while those inside become more adhesive and avillous. This polarity reacts to chemical agents enabling the polar and apolar cells or sections of cells to become visible. The blastomeres now divide transversely at right-angles to the polar axis, giving rise to apolar cells on the inside and polar cells on the outside.[21]

The inner cells divide relatively faster than the larger outer cells that tend to completely cover those inside. During this time desmosomes or glue-like junctions continue to be formed as well as tight junctions. These act as highly selective permeable seals, especially on the outside of the bundle of cells, now called a *morula*, because it looks like a mulberry (Latin *morula*). Gap or communicating junctions are also formed at this time. These allow low-molecular-weight substances to pass by diffusion. Apparently they provide a network for sending inductive signals from cell to cell.[22] This would be essential for various cellular movements and the initial morphological development of cells in early embryos. It seems clear that the polarity associated with the inner and outer cells is related to cell differentiation. It must serve as a prelude to the formation of the ICM and the surrounding trophectoderm cells, both mural and polar.

Gardner gives a clear survey of the early results of experiments on the relevance of cell position in the development of early mouse embryos.[23] It has been found that up to the eight-cell stage all blastomeres can give rise to trophectoderm and that the formation of ICM becomes a possibility for those blastomeres that are on the inside and consequently exposed to more intercellular contacts. When early embryos are aggregated, the outside ones usually, but not exclusively, stay on the outside. There appears to be a strong propensity for the destiny of cells to be influenced by their relative 'inside–outside' position and number of cell contacts. It was found that cells divide asynchronously and that the progeny of the first blastomere to divide at the two-cell stage became more advanced and tended to contribute more than its proportionate share to the formation of the ICM. At least four of the blastomeres of an eight-cell embryo contribute to the ICM and this sometimes occurs after the 16-cell stage, thereby showing a combination of a clear tendency coupled with some flexibility of developmental patterns and potential. Finally, Gardner records that morphogenesis depends on continuous cell interactions and that changes in the density of microvilli, and possibly the extent of contact between blastomeres, may decide whether cells differentiate to become trophectoderm or to form the ICM. These facts do not lend much support to the view that the early embryo is already constituted as the same ontological mammalian individual as the future adult.

Surani and Barton in their research on mouse morulae have provided further evidence to support the thesis that the individual human being could not be present by the morula stage.[24] They were aware there was no extensive mixing of cells in the developing morula, but knew there were some morphogenetic cell movements. These were indicated by tracing in an early morula the relocation of donor cells of different stages of development and taken from various positions in the original morulae. Blastomeres of aggregated morulae could be identified easily by being unlabelled or, alternatively, labelled with fluorescein isothiocynanate.

They were able to confirm that there was a great variation in the number of inner cells, compared to outer cells, for different total populations of cells in embryos that subsequently developed normally. This enabled them to conclude that there must be some dynamic process of cell movement and distribution to adjust the balance of inner and outer blastomeres according to the circumstances. Thus a special dynamic process of various interactions, in addition to the inner and outer spatial distribution of blastomeres, appears to account for the regular constitution and development of morulae prior to the blastocyst stage.

It has been suggested that when the number of inner cells is sufficient, the outer cells are inhibited from dividing and so they spread around the more adhesive and smoother inner cells. Should the number of inner cells be deficient, some of the dividing outer cells join the inner cells until a balance is reached. These varying patterns of behaviour seem to be triggered by differences in the properties of the cell surfaces, especially the more adhesive nature of the surface of the inner cells. This polarization of inner and outer cells varies as they adapt to their changed positions. Cell spreading seems to be incompatible with cell division. It also seems that the inner cells dictate the fate, and control the flexible allocation, of outer blastomeres of the embryo at a stage when their developmental potential or pathway is not yet irreversibly determined, but still dependent on their inner or outer positions. Finally, Surani and Barton suggest that the outer cell that ceased dividing the earliest, positions itself opposite the ICM and becomes the site for the blastocoele formation, thereby marking the site for the abembryonic pole and establishing the embryonic–abembryonic axis.[25]

I think we can conclude from their research that, at the morula stage, it is extremely difficult to establish the presence of the sort of unity that would be required for the cluster of cells to be an actual ontological individual. There does not even appear to be any strict commitment or rigid predetermination in cells from the earliest cleavages to become the inner cells, notwithstanding the probability that the progeny of the first of the two daughter cells of the zygote to divide will contribute more cells to the ICM. The relatively independent behaviour of the individual cells, together with the indeterminate and uncommitted nature of their developmental potential within the cluster of cells as a whole, seems to be incompatible with the individuation of the morula itself as a distinct ontological individual. The flexibility of movement and allocation of cells as distinct entities shown in the whole structure of the morula argues strongly against individuation and personhood from the zygote right up to the morula stage. It is very much like a process involving many individual cells working towards the formation of a greater individual, notwithstanding the presence of a certain element of chance in regard to the timing of early cleavages and the occupation of an inner position by some blastomeres in the morula.

There are signs of finalism or purpose and directedness apparent in the way intercellular communications influence the specific morphogenesis of each species in the same typical way. Developmental activities are goal-directed because they cease when each goal or stage of development is reached. I do not think, however, this would warrant concluding that the morula, after compaction, is already a multicellular individual. Directedness is evident in the various activities and interactions between many living organisms, between male and female animals and humans, and even between sperm and ova themselves, without needing to claim we are dealing with single individuals to account for this sort of purpose and directedness. Directedness and finality are said to be *intrinsic* only if they either appear within, or are adequate evidence of, an already established ontological individual and for its benefit. Quantitative criteria are basic for establishing ontological individuality together with the specific qualitative heterogeneity of an individual's parts. Evidence of the unity of a living individual eutherian mammal should be shown by the nature of the self-maintaining and self-developing activities of a single continuing living body with the same ontological identity. Positive indications are required to establish the presence of a human individual. It would be a vicious circle to argue that something is a living individual on questionable *a priori* grounds that there were *intrinsic* purposive activities. Intrinsic finalism needs to be established and not simply assumed.

3   Parthenogenesis and the human individual

Parthenogenesis refers to the birth of the young without prior sexual intercourse and without the consequent union of the genetic complement of the ovum with that of the male sperm (i.e. virgin birth). It occurs regularly in some vertebrates, such as certain fish and one strain of turkeys, but probably does not naturally or spontaneously occur in any mammal. It has been experimentally induced up to normally developing mid-term gestation in mice with success. Mouse eggs can be activated by manipulative techniques employing the use of alcohol and electric shock to produce haploid and diploid embryos. A parthenogenetic mouse fetus would have to be regarded as an ontological individual and consequently a true mouse at the fetal stage of development so long as it was still alive. Up to that point it develops and grows anatomically the same as any normal mouse. A chimaeric adult mouse can result through the aggregation of a parthenogenetic embryo with a normal mouse embryo.[26] Our knowledge of spontaneous and artificially induced parthenogenetic development of embryos is far from complete. Experimental research on the parthenogenetic development of mouse embryos is presently being pursued with great interest around the world.

Experimental work by McGrath and Solter involving the transplantation of male and female pronuclei between one-cell-stage mouse embryos has given some interesting results.[27] Diploid mouse embryos with two female pronuclei were constructed (biparental gynogenones). Likewise, biparental androgenones were constructed at the single-cell-stage by combining two male pronuclei. The results proved that diploid biparental gynogenetic and androgenetic mouse embryos do not complete normal embryogenesis. The conclusion drawn is that the maternal and paternal genetic contributions to the mammalian embryonic genome are far from being equivalent. A diploid embryo artificially composed of only male or female pronuclei is not capable of sustaining complete embryogenesis. In other words, a mammalian ovum requires the genetic complement of a sperm for normal development to occur beyond the early stages of development.

Research by Surani and his colleagues suggests the maternal chromosomes are more important for the development of a viable embryo proper and fetus, while the paternal chromosomes are more important for the proliferation of healthy extraembryonic membranes and tissues. It is not yet known whether the artificially constructed biparental gynogenetic mouse embryo–fetus is genetically or inherently incapable of developing to full term or whether it simply dies of starvation due to the insufficient development of visceral yolk sac and trophoblast on which the implanted embryo depends for nutrients.[28] This means in practice that both sperm and ovum are required for normal mouse fetal development. The same could be safely said, with our available information, for all eutherian mammals, including humans.

Scientific literature does not report any verification of naturally occurring parthenogenetic development occurring in humans. There is some evidence that a secondary oocyte may begin spontaneous parthenogenetic development at the early cleavage stage, but fails to result in organized development and soon perishes or gives rise to an ovarian teratoma.[29] Some IVF researchers report cases of eight-cell human embryos with only one set of chromosomes (i.e. 23 ×). These would have to be classed as examples of parthenogenetic development of human eggs.[30] For obvious ethical reasons it is not known how far the human parthenogenetic embryo could progress in development either *in vitro* or in the human mother's fallopian tubes or uterus. We cannot accurately extrapolate from the mid-term gestation of the parthenogenetic mouse to the possibility of a human parthenogenetic embryo–fetus.

If we assume that a diploid parthenogenetic human embryo develops normally from the beginning, as in the case of mice, and if completion of fertilization is taken as the beginning of the human being, we would have to conclude that the normally cleaving and developing parthenogenetic human embryo would likewise be a human being until it died. By the same token, the reasons used to argue that the human being does not begin at fertilization would equally apply to argue that the human being does not begin when the human egg is parthenogenetically activated, either spontaneously or artificially. In other words, the phenomenon of parthenogenesis in humans does not *per se* throw any light on the question of when the human individual or person begins. Bear in mind any such hypothetical parthenogenetic human being would be the same as a normal human individual anatomically and physiologically, except for the chromosomes' derivation. These experimental possibilities certainly add to the existing doubts about the completion of fertilization as the beginning of the human individual simply on the grounds of egg activation and the genetic uniqueness that is established at that stage of human development.

4   The human individual not present before completion of implantation

(i)   *Biological facts of the blastocyst stage*

The most crucial transformation to happen to the cleaving cells after fertilization is the formation of the blastocyst, when there are some 60 blastomeres present, some 100 or so hours after fertilization (see Fig. 5.3). The process itself is too well known and documented for there to be any need to go into details beyond what is required for the purposes of this

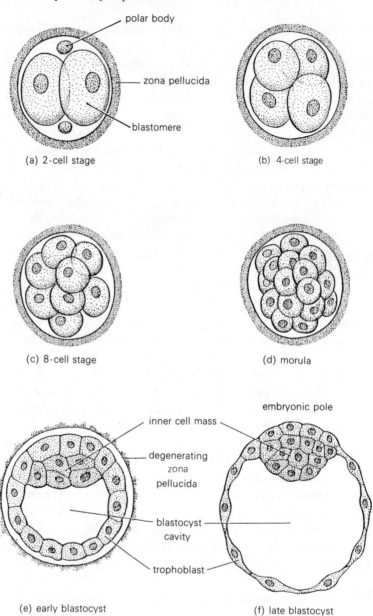

Fig. 5.3. Drawings illustrating cleavage of the zygote and formation of the blastocyst. (*a*)—(*d*) show various stages of cleavage (developmental stage 2). The period of the morula begins at the 12- to 16-cell stage and ends when the blastocyst forms, which occurs when there are 50 to 60 blastomeres present. (*e*) and (*f*) are sections of blastocysts (developmental stage 3). The zona pellucida has disappeared by the late blastocyst stage (five days). The polar

book.[31] The cells of the compacted morula simply begin to differentiate into two broad types of cell, namely, the outer trophectoderm and the ICM. The former proliferate rapidly into mural and polar trophoblast cells that surround the ICM, while the fluid secreted from the cells and the uterine environment accumulates to create the blastocyst cavity or blastocoele. For a couple of days the blastocyst floats freely in the uterine fluid, continuing to exist independently of the mother, but not without some interaction with the uterine environment as the zona pellucida degenerates, allowing the growing blastocyst to hatch out about 140–160 hours after fertilization (see Fig. 5.4).[32]

Over the next week (days 6–13) the process of implantation of the blastocyst in the wall of the womb (i.e. endometrial epithelium) takes place if the natural course of events proceeds smoothly. This results in the formation of the bilaminar embryonic disc from the ICM itself by the start of the second week after fertilization. It consists of the epiblast and hypoblast. The epiblast gives rise to all three germ layers of the embryo, namely, embryonic ectoderm, mesoderm and endoderm. This means that all the cells of the embryo proper are derived from the epiblast alone. Most of the cells originating from the hypoblast probably migrate laterally to form the primitive embryonic endoderm that eventually develops into extraembryonic membranes and tissues. However, a section of the hypoblast thickens to develop into the prochordal plate by day 13–14, indicating the future site of the mouth and serving as an organizer of the head region.[33] Meanwhile, the trophoblast differentiates into two layers – cytotrophoblast and syncytiotrophoblast – as implantation proceeds, establishing the primitive uteroplacental circulation as maternal blood seeps into the lacunar networks. By this time the amniotic cavity has already appeared as a tiny slit between the cytotrophoblast and the ICM. The primary yolk sac is also being formed at this stage, soon to be reduced in size to become the secondary yolk sac.

The timing of blastulation and of the beginning of the process of implantation as well as the minimum number of cells required for successful blastulation is species-specific.[34] If there are too few cells present, blastulation fails due to an insufficient number of cells to form

---

Caption for fig. 5.3 (*cont.*)

bodies shown in (*a*) are small, nonfunctional cells that soon degenerate. (From K. Moore, *The Developing Human: Clinically Oriented Embryology*, Philadelphia: W. B. Saunders Co. 3rd edn, 1982.)

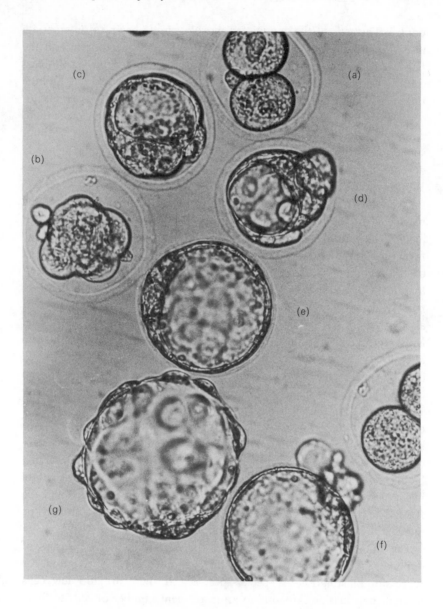

Fig. 5.4. Various stages of development of the mouse embryo that greatly resembles development in the human embryo. (*a*) 2-cell embryo. (*b*) 8-cell embryo at compaction stage. (*c*) Early blastocyst. (*d*) Early blastocyst. See cell being forced out. (*e*) Late or expanded blastocyst. (*f*) Blastocyst hatching out of the zona pellucida. (*g*) Hatched blastocyst. (Reproduced with permission from the editor and authors of *The Journal of Reproduction and Fertility*. Photo – Courtesy Dr A. Trounson.)

both the characteristic species-specific trophectoderm and ICM. By this time the cells would have been reduced to the normal size of somatic cells. The times for cleavage rates and the various stages of embryonic development are fairly similar *in vivo* and *in vitro*, with the latter perhaps being somewhat slower.[35]

As we have already seen, spatial considerations are important in developing the 'inside–outside' polarity of the morula. We also saw that the first of the two original cells to divide contributes a disproportionately large number of progeny to the ICM. These facts, together with the simultaneous blastulation of entire, 'half'- and 'quarter'-embryos have led embryologists to suggest that the timing of early differentiation at the blastocyst stage is governed by some 'clock' mechanism inbuilt into the DNA of the chromosomes of each cell of the embryo. It seems to be set from the time of fertilization, with each cell's 'clock' running in dependence on, and in co-ordination with, what is happening in its surrounding cells.[36]

Development of some cells along one pathway seems to inhibit others from following suit, holding them at bay for the right moment to develop differently. The DNA of the cells seems to resemble minicomputers linked in series for the control of differentiation, development and growth, not only of embryonic life but of all stages of life. It is not known precisely how this 'clock' works beyond that it does so chronologically, controlling growth and development throughout all stages of the life of each individual in conjunction with environmental influences (e.g. freezing practically slows down both clock and development to zero point).[37] If there are too few cells present for any reason, they still attempt to blastulate at the right time, but fail. This is followed by degeneration of the cells.

While in normal circumstances the timing and sequences of developmental stages are set in advance, commitment to one or the other pathway on the part of individual cells is not predetermined, certainly not in any rigid fashion. Reference has been made above to the selective reading of the genetic code of the DNA molecules from the zygote stage on. It must not be thought the code is all read straight through like a book. Lejeune compares the work of reading the information in the DNA to the making of a film.[38] The director selects the sections of film required from kilometres of film footage and clippings. Like an ingenious director, Nature adapts to the circumstances and selects to activate and deactivate at the right time the appropriate genes within the genetically unique chromosomal material available in order to fashion a human individual.

G. C. Liggins makes some interesting observations to fill in the picture:

> Control of cell division and cell differentiation is exerted mainly
> within the tissues themselves by local 'organizers' synthesized
> within the cells in response to genetic information contained in
> their chromosomes. Cells must have a precise mechanism for
> counting replications but its nature in mammalian tissue is
> unknown. In micro-organisms, each cell replication may alter a
> nucleotide in successive codons of a special segment of the DNA
> strand. After a certain number of replications, a codon is reached
> that inhibits further replication when modified.[39]

In some unknown way individual cells are programmed to become
committed to their own pathways (fates), reversible for a while, but
eventually set in a definitive direction of development.

(ii)   *A distinct human individual not formed prior to early differentiation
of the blastocyst*

It would appear that distinct individuation, or the formation of
the cells into a distinct ontological human individual, could not take place
prior to the early blastocyst stage because it is only then that differentiation occurs amongst the cluster of homogeneous cells of the compacted
morula, notwithstanding the 'inside–outside' polarity referred to above. I
do accept that each individual cell is differentiated within itself in relation
to its own heterogeneous parts and that each cell closely resembles the
others at this stage. Not much is understood about why the cells
differentiate into trophectoderm and the ICM when the human blastocyst
is formed.[40] The embryo proper and fetus are derived from the ICM, not
from the trophectoderm, which gives rise to the placenta and extraembryonic membranes.[41] It is very difficult to sustain that the human embryo
could be a human individual prior to the blastocyst stage when it
differentiates into that which will develop into the embryo, fetus and adult
human and that which will not strictly constitute the embryo proper but
will help to sustain such development – the placenta and extraembryonic
membranes. In short, how could the cluster of cells of the early embryo be
an actual ontological human individual if it has not yet differentiated into
the cells and tissues that will constitute the future embryo proper and
those that will not be integral and constituent parts of the embryo proper?

On the other hand, already at this stage could not one begin to think of
the blastocyst as one whole heterogeneous living individual human being?
The structure and properties of the cells of the ICM and trophectoderm

are so different at the blastocyst stage and yet the characteristics and form of each blastocyst are clearly species-specific. Does not this suggest that the blastocyst is already a rudimentary living individual? While both types of cell are so different and both trophectoderm and ICM influence and support each other's separate developmental pathways and growth throughout implantation in a co-ordinated way,[42] I do not think there is sufficient evidence to warrant believing that the blastocyst is already constituted into a distinct human individual with the same ontological identity as the future adult.

Could not the trophoblast and ICM have some organization typical of the blastocyst stage? There is no questioning that extraembryonic tissues, membranes and even the placenta itself are alive and are necessary to protect and/or sustain the developing embryo, but does this mean that they are integral parts of the human embryo proper and eventual fetus itself? How could they be parts of the embryo proper before it is even formed? Bernard Towers considers the placenta and umbilical vessels are living parts of the eventual embryo and fetus that are discarded when no longer needed – somewhat like deciduous teeth.[43] He views the placenta as an extraembryonic organ. But the placenta has no nerves, is insentient and has always been regarded as extraembryonic tissue. While respect and grief have traditionally been expressed for the still-born fetus, at times giving it a burial, this has not been so for the placenta. O'Mahony and Potts observe that in the case of the hydatidiform mole, placental tissue develops without any trace of an embryo at all.[44] This is due to the involvement of only male chromosomes at fertilization (see Fig. 3.1). We have already seen that paternal chromosomes are more important for the formation of extraembryonic tissues, while the maternal chromosomes are more decisive for the development of the embryo proper. All this suggests the placenta, with its less determinate unity and organization, serves as an auxiliary organ for the embryo/fetus to assist in performing its functions of nutrition, respiration and excretion, but not that it is formally an integral constituent part of the embryo/fetus itself. In the case of identical twins, one placenta may serve the needs of two distinct fetuses but it would not formally be a constituent part of either twin fetus. Maternal organs are also indispensible for the survival and support of the embryo/fetus, but they are not constituent parts of the embryo/fetus itself.

The constant and universal organic pattern of the blastocyst, its heterogeneous differentiation and developmental pathways are certainly purposive and goal directed. It displays a certain teleological plan inbuilt in its organic dynamism as development in the formation of a human individual proceeds closer to realization. No matter how we describe the blastocyst's cohesion, for the reason given above it does not seem to be the same living human individual that is about to actually begin. The same thing could also be said of the zygote, at a stage further removed. The blastocyst does not seem to be the same ontological individual as the future adult human individual. Whatever unity is had at the blastocyst stage, it does not appear to be the ontological unity of a distinct human individual that is retained throughout all subsequent stages of development to birth and beyond. The teleological system of the blastocyst should not be identified with the ontological unity of the human individual that will develop from it.

(iii)   *Animal experiments show insufficient actual determination of the late blastocyst to be a distinct individual*

At the early pre-implantation stages cells can develop into either embryonic or extraembryonic lineages – i.e. they are not yet definitively committed or determined to form the embryo proper. This broad embryological potency of cells displayed during the early cleavage stages becomes gradually restricted, but not totally eliminated, at the blastocyst stage, as we have already noted when referring to the possibility of identical twinning within single blastocysts. If they are damaged, they are able to recuperate perfectly and resume normal development. The ICM is able to induce the polar trophoblast cells to proliferate and provide more mural and giant trophoblast cells until implantation has occurred. Blastocysts can survive when large parts of the ICM are destroyed. At late blastocyst differentiation, the cells of the ICM and trophectoderm enter upon mutually exclusive pathways of development. There is ample evidence to support this fact by the expanded blastocyst stage.[45] Cell determination does not necessarily imply, however, that the individual human being is already constituted.

Experiments on blastocysts suggest the late blastocyst could not yet be regarded as an individual mouse, sheep or human being. As we have already seen, experiments with sheep show that blastulation occurs at the same time with entire, half- and quarter-embryos with decreasing success rates respectively. This would seem to indicate that for blastulation to occur successfully, compaction should already have taken place and the minimum species-specific number of 'inner' and 'outer' cells should be present at the time predetermined for blastulation to occur. This is pre-set from the moment of fertilization in the 'clock' of the DNA in each cell that is produced. This suggests a gradual process precedes not only blastulation, but also the transformation of a group or system of co-ordinated individual cells into a multicellular heterogeneous living individual human being, capable of retaining the same ontological identity throughout all subsequent stages of development. This seems to accord more with the facts and would obviate the difficulties involved in maintaining that the fertilized egg itself is a human being that retains the same personal identity throughout successive cleavages and developmental stages.

Gardner's experiments with reconstituted mouse blastocysts seem to confirm the thesis that the blastocyst itself has not yet become the same multicellular individual that retains a continuing ontological identity beyond birth to the adult stage. He devised techniques to separate trophectoderm and ICM tissues in blastocysts. He proceeded to transfer donor ICM tissues to host trophectoderm that lacked polar trophectoderm and found that more than half developed into normal fetuses after successful implantations. The genetic markers used showed that trophoblast was derived only from the trophectoderm, while the fetus, amnion, allantois and yolk sac were derived from the donor ICM. This means a normal fetus can develop when surrounded by genetically different trophoblast and extraembryonic membranes and tissues. Similar results have been obtained involving work to produce inter-species chimaerism. Goat ICM cells have been injected into expanded sheep blastocysts of the same age as the goat embryos from which the ICM cells were removed. Of the nine live offspring born to the recipient female sheep, two were overt sheep–goat chimaeras and one was a pure goat kid.[46] Trophectoderm alone, without any ICM cells, soon ceases to develop and cannot give rise to a living fetus: together they harmoniously succeed.

Consideration of this evidence leads one to conclude that if ICM and trophectodermal cells, taken from blastocysts of the same or different species, can be aggregated to enable an embryo proper and a viable fetus to develop, surely this is a sign that normal trophectodermal and ICM cells, derived from the progeny of the same zygote, likewise follow the same developmental pattern. This would certainly confirm the view that the normal blastocyst is really a goal-directed system of heterogeneous cells, but not yet a definitive multicellular heterogeneous living individual member of a mammalian species – human or otherwise.

Gardner describes more experiments using clonal analysis of development to show that individual cells from a mouse ICM can be injected into host mouse blastocysts to trace their fate. It was shown that single donor cells from a three-and-a-half-day ICM could contribute progeny to all the tissues of the conceptus that normally derive from the ICM of an intact

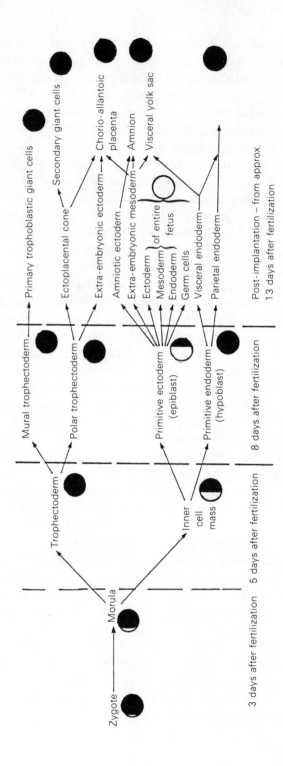

Fig. 5.5. Presumptive scheme of cell lineages in the early human embryo based on transplantation of genetically marked mouse cells and tissues into blastocysts. Restriction in developmental potential can be clearly seen. Shaded sections of circles represent one or more cells from which will develop extraembryonic tissues. Unshaded sections represent cell(s) from which will develop the entire embryo proper and fetus. Adapted from C. R. Austin and R. V. Short, *Embryonic and Fetal Development*, *Reproduction in Mammals*, Bk. 2, Cambridge: C.U.P., 1982.

blastocyst. This is a sign that the relatively undifferentiated cells of the ICM of an early blastocyst are fairly unrestricted in their developmental potential for all the tissues of the entire fetus as well as for some extraembryonic endoderm. The case is different with the four-and-a-half-day ICM cells that are already differentiated into epiblast (primitive ectoderm) and hypoblast (primitive endoderm). The primitive endoderm clones contribute progeny to one or both the extraembryonic membranes, while the primitive ectoderm clones contribute progeny throughout the whole fetus, including the amnion, allantois and the mesodermal layer of the yolk sac too. The testing of these chimaeras has shown that these primitive ectoderm clones contribute to the germ-cell line as well as to the rest of the mouse soma and some extraembryonic mesoderm. Primitive endoderm clones are restricted to extraembryonic endoderm alone.[47]

As a result of all this work, fairly comprehensive fate maps can be drawn showing the details of location of the various derivatives of the trophectoderm and the ICM (see Fig. 5.5).[48] The trophectoderm eventually contributes cells to the primary and secondary giant cells and the chorio–allantoic placenta. The ICM differentiates into the epiblast from which are chiefly derived, after implantation, the ectoderm, the mesoderm and the endoderm of the entire fetus. The ICM also gives origin to the hypoblast which develops into the primitive endoderm, from which are derived visceral and parietal endoderm. This shows that the late blastocyst is far from being sufficiently differentiated and determined in itself, in relation to the future embryo proper, before the completion of implantation by the end of the second week. In other words, before a person can be present or formed, we need to have an actually distinct, determined and undivided individual whose ontological identity continues unchanged until the adult stage – not one that is still only potential and indeterminate. Experiments with chimaeric blastocysts show that this could hardly occur before the late blastocyst stage.

There is no evidence to suggest that all of a sudden, as though by magic, individual cells become a human individual. While each cell develops following its own encoded programme, this is not done independently of its neighbouring cells. They influence each other and together form groups that differentiate in similar ways to become various types of specialized cell tissues and eventually organ primordia. Groups of cells become committed to various pathways as though the actualization of their natural developmental potential was triggered by random encounters and chance events, always within defined limits. The natural totipotency of the early cleavage cells is gradually restricted and lost as they journey along their own pathways. Natural totipotency gradually passes from each cell of the early cleavage stage to groups of cells from the morula or from the ICM. Further down the developmental track, totipotency is possessed only by larger segments of entire blastocysts. In this way the developmental potential and independence of behaviour of individual cells are gradually restricted before the eventual formation of the definitive human individual. This certainly indicates a gradual formation of the human individual through various stages from undifferentiated and indeterminate individual early cleavage cells to heterogeneous groups of cells or tissues as cell multiplication and differentiation progress. A determinate, actual human individual gradually emerges and develops from what is potentially human and indeterminate in relation to its ultimate fate. This does not mean any particular cell is not determined with respect to what it actually is at any stage of development.

One could ask would it not be enough for the ICM to differentiate into the epiblast, the hypoblast and the prochordal plate for one to reasonably maintain that an individual human being was formed? The prochordal plate and the epiblast still seem to be discrete, separate tissues or groups of cells that are interacting with each other.[49] Certainly not much more would be needed for individuation to be achieved. The indication of the site of the mouth alone would not constitute a body plan and would seem to need the complementary individuation provided by the arrival of the primitive streak itself, if there is to be a distinct individual human being that continues with the same ontological identity from that time onwards. In fact, the primitive streak appears shortly afterwards, if not about the same time on day 14. The unity of the individual human organism would imply a characteristic minimal specific heterogeneity of quantitative parts arranged to provide determinate sites for the co-ordinated development of structures, tissues and organs along a primordial body axis. This would not seem to have been achieved with the mere appearance of the prochordal plate. We are not dealing with arbitrary requirements: they are determined by the concept of person we all employ. This concept, in its turn, is based on our direct experience and ordinary understanding of individual human persons, complemented by reflection on this original experience in the light of metaphysical principles.

It has also been found that cells from the primitive ectoderm of post-implantation mouse embryos could successfully colonize blastocysts, while those derived from the trophectodermal and primitive endodermal derivatives were unable to do so.[50] This shows that whilst the developmental potential of the post-implantation primitive ectodermal derivatives still persisted, that of trophectodermal and primitive endodermal derivatives was restricted. We might recall that the embryo proper and fetus derive from the cells of the primitive ectoderm. This could very well mean that the post-implantation trophectodermal and primitive endodermal derivatives of the human embryos are likewise restricted in their developmental potential. In turn, this suggests that the threshold for the formation of the human individual is shortly after implantation.

I do not think any firm conclusions can be drawn from these experiments to establish the precise time when a human embryo is actually individualized to become a human individual as distinct from having only the potential to become a human being. I think arguments based on the totipotency of cells or blastocysts alone cannot provide the complete solution to our problem, even if they may be helpful. Some more positive indication is required. A multicellular individual is actually to be a human individual, not simply something that has the potential to become a human individual. Whatever is only a potential human individual cannot yet be an actual individual human person.

On the other hand, loss of totipotency could be significant for establishing when an actual individual human being has been formed. The stage when parts of a blastocyst or developing embryo lose their totipotency could indicate that their potential is restricted precisely because species-specific individuation has already occurred, i.e. when a distinct multicellular individual has already been formed, endowed with heterogeneous parts for its structures, organs and tissues. Once an actual human individual is formed, the potential to form one or more individuals would no longer be needed by the developing cells and tissues. Still some positive sign of the formation of a distinct individual would be required. In the final chapter we shall see if there are any grounds for drawing a line at some stage in the developmental process before which it is not likely that a human individual could be present, or after which stage most likely, or most certainly, a human individual would already be formed.

6

The human individual begins after implantation

1   Distinctive development of eutherian mammalian embryos

The use of experimental methods to increase knowledge of the early stages of eutherian mammalian development had to wait until the middle of the twentieth century. Mammals are viviparous and consequently their embryos could not survive for long outside the uterine environment until the techniques of tissue culture became available. Much progress has been made over the last 30 years. Perhaps in the future it will become possible for a mouse embryo to develop to term artificially outside the womb. For the present, early mammalian embryology might better be termed 'pre-embryology' since it concentrates more on the formation of the extraembryonic membranes. These develop during the preimplantation stage and provide support and nutrition for the embryo proper that is only formed subsequently. The case of amphibian embryos is quite different because they do not need extraembryonic membranes, the placenta in particular.[1] It has been relatively easy to study their developmental stages from the start right through to term. Accordingly, it would be quite misleading to apply to the development of eutherian mammalian embryos what properly applies only to amphibian embryos.

Regionalization and symmetry begin soon after fertilization in monospermic amphibians like frogs and toads. The grey crescent appears in the animal pole opposite the point of entry of the sperm and marks the future dorsal side of the amphibian. The first cleavage is vertical and divides the egg into right and left halves. The next cleavage is at right-angles to the first and separates the ventral and dorsal halves. The third cleavage is equatorial and separates the animal and vegetal halves (see Fig. 6.1). It is clear that important decisions for the body plan of such amphibians are made at fertilization itself.[2]

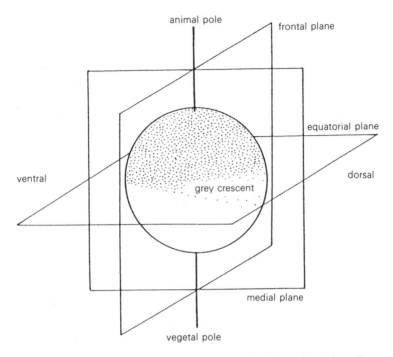

Fig. 6.1. Axes of the amphibian egg after fertilization. (Reproduced from *From Egg to Embryo: Determinative Events in Early Development*, by J. M. W. Slack with the permission of Cambridge University Press, 1983.)

On the other hand, regional specification and symmetry of the body plan in the eutherian mammalian embryo does not take place early in development. We have seen in the mouse, sheep and human that it does not occur until after implantation when embryonic and extraembryonic tissues have been fairly well segregated and the proliferating and differentiating cells have passed the threshold of no return in their various developmental pathways.[3] In this way the totipotency and pluripotency of the individual cells and groups of cells is gradually restricted as cell commitment is established. No evidence has been found in mammalian embryos of the presence of localized organizer regions that are so characteristic and determining for the developmental pathways in the amphibian zygote and early embryo, e.g. the animal and vegetal pole (see Fig. 6.1).[4] Unlike mammals, identical twinning can only take place in amphibians if the axis of cleavage of the zygote leaves the right cytoplasmic contents in each blastomere (see Fig 6.2).[5]

Even after externally induced random movements or disaggregation of

CLEAVAGE IN AMPHIBIANS

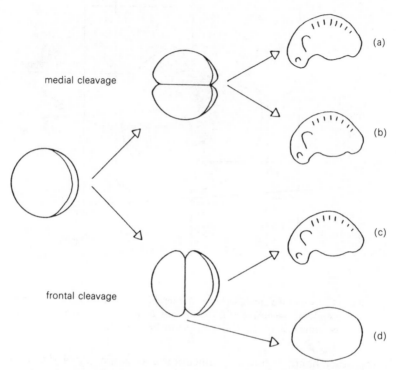

Fig. 6.2. Production of twins by separation of the first two blastomeres. If cleavage occurs in the medial plane both blastomeres produce an embryo (*a, b*). If cleavage occurs in the frontal plane the ventral blastomere can produce a symmetrical 'belly piece' (*c, d*). (Reproduced from *From Egg to Embryo: Determinative Events in Early Development* by J. M. W. Slack, with the permission of Cambridge University Press, 1983.)

cells, orderly development towards the formation of the embryo proper and fetus usually resumes with early mammalian embryos and blastocysts. When a cell lineage forks, frequently one line continues on a pathway for further differentiation within a set of given possibilities, while the other terminates differentiation to maintain a particular type of cell tissue, according to need, by synthesizing the same proteins (see Fig. 6.3). This is done by some genes remaining switched-on and others switched-off. Somatic cells differ because they express different genes, even though all

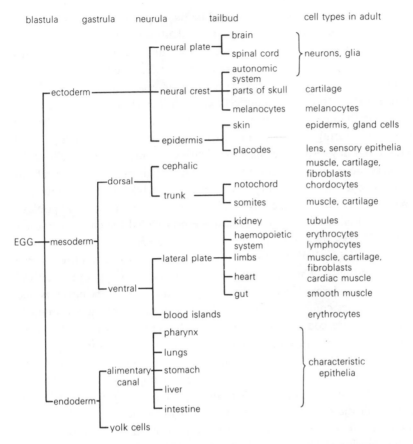

Fig. 6.3. Formation of the basic body plan in a vertebrate (excluding extra-embryonic regions). By the early tailbud stage the embryo consists of a mosaic of regions determined to form the principal organs and structures of the body. This body plan is built up as a result of a hierarchy of decisions, and several further decisions will in most cases be taken before the cells differentiate into the terminal cell types shown on the right-hand side. It should be noted that some cell types, such as cartilage, arise from more than one lineage. (Reproduced from *From Egg to Embryo: Determinative Events in Early Development*, by J. M. W. Slack, with the permission of Cambridge University Press, 1983.)

the genes are found in every cell. Mammalian development depends on mechanical, biochemical and electric inductive signals between cells, whose developmental potency is thereby triggered and activated to gradually form a morula, an implanted blastocyst, an embryo proper, a fetus and a live offspring after birth (see Fig. 6.3).

2   **The human individual formed by the stage of gastrulation**

It is time to attempt a positive identification of when a human individual begins with some degree of certitude. In practice this means examining the embryological facts to find out when the epiblast (primitive ectoderm) ceases to be a cluster of more or less homogeneous cells to differentiate into a single multicellular, heterogeneous developing living human individual. There are strong, almost compelling, reasons to believe this occurs during the process of gastrulation that begins about day 14 and ends about day 19 after fertilization. During this process some cells of the epiblast break away and form the mesoblast. This provides some cells to form a layer of intraembryonic mesoderm, while others become the embryonic endoderm, thereby displacing some cells from the hypoblast. The cells that are left in the epiblast are now called the embryonic ecto- derm (see Figs. 5.5 and 6.4). The cells of these three layers divide, differen- tiate, develop and grow into the tissues and organs of the entire embryo proper and fetus. The outer epithelia and the nervous system are derived from the ectoderm. The epithelial linings of the respiratory passages and digestive tract come from the endoderm. The mesoderm gives origin to smooth muscle coats, connective tissues, blood cells, bone marrow, the skeleton and the reproductive and excretory organs (see Fig. 6.3).[6]

Development is continuous throughout the third week. The neural plate makes its appearance during this week, developing into the neural groove by day 18, with the neural folds beginning to move together and fuse by the end of the same week, soon to give origin to the neural tube. This is important for it means that the formation of the central nervous system that comprises the brain and the spinal cord has made significant progress by 21 days after fertilization. By the same time the endocardial heart tubes have developed and begun to fuse into the primitive heart tube. By day 21 the circulation of blood has almost certainly begun, linking up blood vessels in the embryo, the connecting stalk, the chorion and the yolk sac. This means that the cardiovascular system is the first organ to begin functioning, supplying nutrients for the benefit of the whole newly formed developing human organism (see Appendix II).[7]

This fact, together with the constitution of the primordium of the central nervous system (neural plate, groove and finally tube) provides fairly convincing evidence that after the third week a single, biologically human, whole heterogeneous individual living organism already exists, functioning and developing as one continuing ontological individual. This would be an individual with a human nature. I find it difficult to doubt that the same tiny human organism, three weeks after fertilization,

GASTRULATION

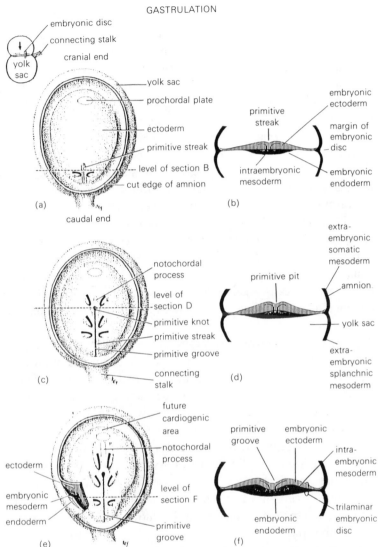

Fig. 6.4. Drawings illustrating formation of the trilaminar embryonic disc (developmental stage 6, days 15 to 16). The small sketch at the upper left is for orientation; the arrow indicates the dorsal aspect of the embryonic disc as shown in (*a*). The arrows in all other drawings indicate migration of mesenchymal cells between the ectoderm and endoderm. (*a*), (*c*) and (*e*), Dorsal views of the embryonic disc early in the third week, exposed by removal of the amnion. (*b*), (*d*) and (*f*), Transverse sections through the embryonic disc at the levels indicated. The prochordal plate is indicated by a broken line because it is a thickening of endoderm that cannot be seen from the dorsal surface. (From K. Moore, *The Developing Human: Clinically Oriented Embryology*, Philadelphia: W. B. Saunders, 1982, with slight modifications from colour to black and white.)

continues to grow and develop with the same ontological identity as the baby that is subsequently born and matures as an adult human individual.

It is not essential that all organs be present and functioning. It would be a sufficient, but probably not a necessary, condition for an individual human being to exist that it be a living body with the primordium of at least one organ formed for the benefit of the whole organism. The fact that nutrients are received now directly from the mother and enable the *embryo as a whole to grow* signifies that a new on-going living ontological individual has been formed. In order to retain the same ontological individual human identity throughout all stages of growth, it would be necessary for all the organs that are formed to be integrated into one central organization and function for the benefit of the one whole living individual. Obviously I do not believe the genetic code in the DNA of the genes of the zygote could be taken as the equivalent of an organ of a human being. The genetic instructions for the formation of the whole human being and its organs must not be confused with the actual human being and its organs. Again I appeal to the concept of real existence and of a human individual that we actually employ in our conceptual scheme.

3   The human individual begins at the primitive streak stage

I have argued that after gastrulation, by the end of the third week when the neural folds have been formed and the primitive cardiovascular system is functioning to enable nutrition and growth as a whole to take place, there are sufficient reasons to justify asserting that a living individual with a human nature has been formed. Consequently, a human being or person is present. The question arises whether these activities represent only the sufficient, or also the necessary, conditions for having a human individual. In other words, can a good case be made out for a human individual beginning after the blastocyst stage and the completion of implantation but before the end of the third week? I shall now attempt to answer this question.

Before gastrulation begins there is a cluster or assemblage of a few thousand cells that constitute the epiblast, from which there will eventually be derived the entire ectoderm, mesoderm and endoderm of the developing embryo proper and fetus. These are the only cells that are not destined to become part of extraembryonic tissues. I have already observed that they appear to lack the requisite organic unity to constitute a single individual at the end of implantation, i.e. about day 13. As gastrulation is getting under way, however, at about day 14–15, a convergence of epiblastic cells occurs in the posterior part of the

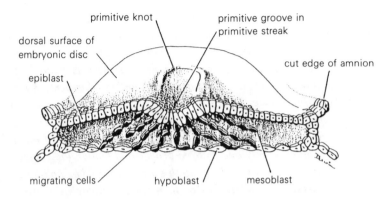

dorsal surface of
embryonic disc

primitive knot

epiblast

primitive groove in
primitive streak

cut edge of amnion

migrating cells   hypoblast   mesoblast

Fig. 6.5. Drawing of the cranial half of the embryonic disc during the third week. The disc has been cut transversely to show the migration of mesenchymal cells from the primitive streak. This illustration also indicates that the definitive embryonic endoderm probably also arises from the epiblast. Presumably, the hypoblastic cells are displaced to extraembryonic regions. (From K. Moore, *The Developing Human: Clinically Oriented Embryology*, Philadelphia: W. B. Saunders, 1982, with slight modifications from colour to black and white.)

embryonic disc: this is called the primitive streak. It is a key factor, a primary organizer for the process of differentiation during gastrulation. It gradually elongates and thickens as cells pile up to form the primitive knot, the primitive groove and the primitive pit (see Figs. 6.4, 6.5 and Appendix II).

Usually the cells piling up on the embryonic plate form only one primitive streak. Sometimes none is formed, with the result that no embryo proper develops, but only a 'blighted ovum' with no potential to form an embryo proper. The primitive streak might fail to appear on account of a deficiency of epiblast cells in the embryonic plate. Some cells from the epiblast do not form part of the embryo proper, but contribute to the formation of the allantois which combines with extraembryonic mesoblast to form the umbilical cord. By this stage, some 16 days after fertilization, all the cells derived from the zygote have been committed to being part of extraembryonic structures or part of the embryo proper. Only very rarely do the cells form two primitive streaks, from which live identical twins may develop. This is the last stage at which identical twins may be formed.[8]

The appearance of the primitive streak is an important landmark, indicating the position of the embryo proper with the main features of the new individual's body plan. *This appears to be the stage of development when the cells of the epiblast first become organized through this primitive streak into one whole multicellular individual living human being, possessing for the first time a body axis and bilateral symmetry. Its developing cells are now integrated and subordinated to form a single heterogeneous organic body that endures with its own ontological as well as biological identity through all its subsequent stages of growth and development. A new human individual begins once the matter of the epiblastic cells becomes one living body, informed or actuated by a human form, life-principle or soul that arises through the creative power of God. The appearance of one primitive streak signals that only one embryo proper and human individual has been formed and begun to exist. Prior to this stage it would be pointless to speak about the presence of a true human being in an ontological sense. A human individual could scarcely exist before a definitive human body is formed. As mentioned earlier, the formation of an ontological individual with a truly human nature and rational ensoulment must coincide.*

We should recall that the cell derivatives of the primitive endoderm from post-implantation mouse embryos fail to colonize host blastocysts to form chimaeras. By that stage their development along specific pathways is irreversible, no longer having the potential to return to the pluripotency typical of the blastocyst stage. There is every reason to believe the same principle applies in post-implantation human embryos, especially after the appearance of the primitive streak.[9] Developmental potential is restricted in these cells because they are committed to specific regions or parts of the extraembryonic endoderm. Once particular sites or positions within the definitive growing embryo become designated for the development of specific structures, systems and organs, it is a sign that an on-going multicellular ontological human individual has already been formed and actually exists. Organogenesis can only start once defined regions of the heterogeneous individual human body become allocated for the development of specific structures and organs. Potency for differentiation, development and growth can only be actualized through this regional specification. Without this, I fail to see how an actual individual human being could be present. This would be a condition required to pass from the presence of a potential human individual to an actual human individual with potential.

Once the primitive streak stage is passed, it is already determined whether there will be one or two definitive embryos formed. If only one streak appears, regional specification involving pattern formation and spatial organization of symmetry immediately becomes actualized. These broad developmental decisions are biologically irreversible. This is why after this stage the potency for identical twinning is lost. A part of the embryo proper, even half of it, cannot resume the process of regional specification to form another individual embryo proper. In short, the potency for identical twinning is lost after the primitive streak stage because an actual human individual has already been formed. The potency is lost because there are no more cells or groups of cells there developing to become one or more human individuals. That threshold has already been irrevocably passed once a human individual is formed. Unlike the bacterial cell, the amoeba or the zygote, a human individual does not have the potency to give rise to identical twins through division. Our constant experience shows that cutting a human individual in two simply kills that individual.

One who holds the view that the human individual begins at the zygote stage could in theory suggest that the embryonic human individual has the potency to form identical twins up to the primitive streak stage. In this respect the embryonic human individual would be compared to the bacterial cell or the amoeba. But this theoretical possibility fails, as we have already seen, for lack of evidence to show that the zygote is a human individual. One cannot argue deductively that the human individual may twin any time between the zygote stage and the primitive streak stage when one has simply assumed *a priori* that the zygote already is an actual human individual in the first place. The use of inductive philosophical reasoning leads to the conclusion that the human individual begins at the primitive streak stage, but not before it. This is so because the conditions for the presence of an actual human individual, in the sense of an on-going living ontological individual with a true human nature, are not satisfied prior to the formation of the primitive streak.

In very rare instances two primitive streaks may be formed that give rise to identical twins, even conjoined or Siamese twins. Such an exceptional case would not affect the validity of the conclusions reached above. Prior to the formation of the two primitive streaks, there would not yet be any human individual formed at all. Two human individuals would originate from the amalgamating heterogeneous cells as they form two primitive streaks. Conjoined twins result if the two streaks are not completely separated, but are partly joined. In other words, two human individuals would arise from a specifically heterogeneous mass of epiblastic cells that had the developmental potency to form one or more than one human individual.[10] The fact that some conjoined twins share some limbs or even vital organs does not mean two human individuals have not been formed. If two complete human heads are formed, it is commonly accepted two human individuals are formed. When there is one complete head and four legs we assume there is only one human individual, one subject of rational and free acts, not two. For the same reason there would be one human individual if there were two partially formed heads sharing one brain. Certainly these cases highlight the fact that human individuals come into existence by a process, a process that lasts about two weeks instead of a day or the moment the sperm penetrates the egg.

Keith Moore succinctly expresses the significance of the primitive streak in embryological terms:

> When the primitive streak appears, it is possible to identify the embryo's craniocaudal axis, its cranial and caudal ends, its dorsal and ventral surfaces, and its right and left sides.[11]

Given the right conditions regarding the minimum number of epiblastic cells, environmental factors and the passing of the species-specific length of time from fertilization, the individual cells and different tissues are able to follow up their reciprocal communication signals by interacting to coalesce and form a new and greater individual living body. It now has a characteristic property of an individual body that did not exist previously. There is a definite spatial determination within the one body for the development of the different organs required for growth, self-maintenance and eventual reproduction. When this distinct individuation occurs, there arises the fundamental craniocaudal axis for the basic internal disposition of organs and parts that practically remain unchanged for the entire life of the individual. The basic body plan of the human individual is normally definitively determined for life at this stage.

Anne McLaren in discussing this same question comes to a conclusion quite similar to my own concerning the beginning of the human individual:

> The primitive streak stage is a vitally important landmark in development because it marks the onset of *individuality*. ... once the primitive streak has formed, we can for the first time recognise and delineate the boundaries of a discrete coherent entity, an individual, that can become transformed through growth and differentiation into an adult human being. If I had to point to a stage and say 'This was when I began being me', I think it would have to be here.[12]

Subsequently she expressed her views in more detail:

> If we are talking not about the origin of life ... but about the origin of an individual life, one can trace back directly from the

newborn baby to the foetus, and back further to the origin of the individual embryo at the primitive streak stage in the embryonic plate at sixteen or seventeen days. If one tries to trace back further than that there is no longer a coherent entity. Instead there is a larger collection of cells, some of which are going to take part in the subsequent development of the embryo and some of which aren't.[13]

Prior to this stage we do not have a living individual human body, but a mass of pre-programmed loosely organized developing cells and heterogeneous tissues until their 'clock' mechanisms become synchronized and triggered to harmoniously organize, differentiate and grow as heterogeneous parts of a single whole human organism. In this way the cells lose their own ontological individuality to form a new ontological individual.[14] This change enables many actual individual cells and tissues to realize their potential to become a new multicellular developing human individual with a human nature. I think the sort of individuation and multicellular unity displayed with the appearance of the primitive streak justifies the claim that this is the beginning of an individual being that is a human person with the potential to develop to the age of reason. As I have argued earlier, the human individual would be ensouled from its beginning at the primitive streak stage with a rational soul or life-principle since it is the form of the human body, i.e. it makes the human body be the same individual from that stage until death. Being a non-material or spiritual soul, there could not be any direct empirical evidence for its presence prior to the age of reason.

Once the human individual has been formed at the primitive streak stage, the development of organs or organogenesis soon begins. Not so much individual cells, but groups of cells within the embryo, now become successively committed to form specific tissues or organs in an orderly way within the embryo proper during the following six weeks.[15] Fetal development then continues until the baby is born (see Appendixes II and III).

I have come to the same conclusions as Dr J. J. Diamond who first set my mind in this direction many years ago, though I did not find his original presentation of the arguments convincing. I believe I have uncovered sufficient biological evidence to justify his conclusions:

... when the organiser appears in the cell mass, it is irrevocably determined that the unity of the individual is established; for twinning can no longer occur and reconjunction can no longer occur ... the metaphysician ... cannot possibly entertain the notion of ensoulment prior to the point where it is biologically established that either one or several human entities have resulted from fertilization ... there is a point earlier than which ensoulment cannot be held to be infused, which point lies at that stage of the gestational biology where the individuality of the entity is irrevocably laid down in the nature of things ... I submit that we can justifiably hold that at fertilization is laid down *only* the characteristic of the subsequently hominizable entity(ies), the hominization and individualization of which cannot be posited until the late-second or early-third week after fertilization.[16]

My conclusions are likewise in broad agreement with those of John Mahoney who has recently discussed this question:

> Only the conclusions to be drawn from the facts of actual or possible twinning and combination of fertilised eggs appear to resist critical examination and to indicate that, rather than ensoulment occurring at the stage of conception, it can take place only when there is an unambiguously individual subject capable of receiving the soul by virtue of the fact that it is passing beyond the stage of simple reduplication and is beginning to ramify and diversify through the development of its bodily organs.[17]

Without committing himself in the matter, Paul Ramsey clearly admits the force of the arguments in favour of human individuation beginning only after identical twinning or segmentation could no longer take place:

> It might be asserted that it is at the time of segmentation, not earlier, that life comes to be the individual human being it is ever thereafter to be....

> If there is a moment in the development of these nascent lives of ours subsequent to fertilization and prior to birth (or graduation from college) at which it would be reasonable to believe that an individual human life begins and therefore begins to be inviolate, that moment is arguably at the stage when segmentation may or may not take place.[18]

Perhaps the persons most concerned in human reproduction can offer some valuable information from their own experience. Nature's own sign to a woman that she may be pregnant is her first missed menses after sexual intercourse. This would usually occur about two weeks after fertilization. This is the time when the primitive streak would have appeared after implantation had taken place. This is why some biologists suggest that we should regard implantation itself as conception. In suggesting this, there would be a return to the original meaning of conception, of a woman becoming pregnant by holding or taking to herself the *seed* that has become an embryo, 'the growing one'.

4   Significance of government reports

The Warnock Committee did not enter the philosophical arena by attempting to establish when a human being begins. Its task was to make recommendations to Parliament concerning the social, ethical and legal implications of recent and potential developments in the field of human assisted reproduction.[19] Its account of embryological facts and development is eminently descriptive in empirical terms. It did admit in its Report that once the reproductive process had begun:

> ... there is no particular part of the developmental process that is more important than another; all are part of a continuous process, and unless each stage takes place normally, at the correct time, and in the correct sequence, further development will cease. Thus biologically there is no single identifiable stage in the development of the embryo beyond which the *in vitro* embryo should not be kept alive.[20]

The Report also noted that in the embryonic disc:

> ... the first recognisable features of the embryo proper will appear. The first of these features is the primitive streak, which appears as a heaping up of cells at one end of the embryonic disc on the fourteenth or fifteenth day after fertilisation ... This is the latest stage at which identical twins can occur.[21]

Finally the Warnock Report says:

> One reference point in the development of the human individual is the formation of the primitive streak. Most authorities put this at about 15 days after fertilisation. This marks the beginning of individual development of the embryo.[22]

The *Waller Report* to the Victorian Government is similar to the *Warnock Report* in its scope and purpose but does not go into the embryological details to the same extent.[23] It does not employ the concepts of 'individuation' and 'personhood'. It uses the term 'entity' in a general or non-technical sense when it refers to the embryo as 'an individual and genetically unique human entity',[24] or 'an independent and unique human entity', without adopting any philosophical position in relation to its meaning or unity.[25] It refers to:

> ... the stage of implantation, which is completed 14 days after fertilization. It is after this stage that the primitive streak is formed, and differentiation of the embryo is clearly evident.[26]

It is significant that both the above Reports, among other things, recommend the banning of experimentation on human embryos beyond the 14-day limit, even if this research is deemed necessary for the advancement of medical knowledge and therapies.[27] Such legislation was deemed necessary out of regard for our common moral sense and respect for human embryos as well as to allay the publicly expressed fears and concern of the community in this delicate matter. More importantly, I am inclined to believe the members of both the Warnock and the Waller Committees felt that beyond 14 days after fertilization, when normally implantation and the formation of the primitive streak would have taken place, the developing individual embryo commands the respect of all. For the members of the Warnock Committee this was so because of the embryo's *individuation at the primitive streak stage*, while for the members of the Waller Committee it was the *clearly evident differentiation that follows the primitive streak stage*. For both Committees the formation of the primitive streak was extremely significant in terms of the legally enforceable respect due to the developing human embryo.

Baroness Warnock has since confirmed my hunch concerning the significance of the primitive streak for the Warnock Committee. As chairman of the Committee she is quite qualified to interpret the reasons underlying its recommendations:

> We, the majority of the Inquiry, recommend that research on the human embryo should be brought to an end on the fourteenth day because of the development then of the primitive streak. Up to that time, it is difficult to think of the embryo as an individual, because it might still become two individuals. None of the criteria of identity that apply to me, or Tom or Dick or Harry, and distinguish one of us from the others, are satisfied by the embryo at this very early stage. The collection of cells, though loosely strung together, is hardly yet one thing, nor is it several. It is not yet determined to be either one or several. But from the fourteenth or fifteenth day onwards, there is no doubt that it is Tom or Dick or Harry that is developing, or all three of them, but as three individuals. At this stage, then, the embryo proper has

become distinct from those cells which will become its protective cover in the uterus, the placenta. Up to this time as I have said the whole collection of cells may be thought of, not as an embryo, but as a pre-embryo.[28]

The Australian *Senate Select Committee on the Human Embryo Experimentation Bill 1985* concluded differently for after fertilization:

> ... the embryo may be properly described as genetically new human life organized as a distinct entity oriented towards further development ... of a biologically individuated member of the human species.[29]

It must be admitted this is normally true, except in the case where chromosomal changes may occur in the developing embryo subsequent to the formation of the zygote.[30] It should be noted that the reference to 'a biologically individuated member of the human species' does not necessarily imply the zygote is a continuing ontologically distinct individual member of the human species. We have already emphasized that 'genetic individuality' and 'ontological individuality' are not the same thing. After the primitive streak stage when identical twinning can no longer take place, the human embryo is definitively both a biologically and ontologically individuated member of the human species or a human individual. As we have already seen, the Senate Committee did not attempt 'to attribute the status of "person" to the embryo either in its philosophical or legal senses' (see above, p. 6).

Great significance is given to the empirically verifiable genetic discontinuity that occurs at fertilization when a genetically unique embryo is constituted. Implantation and the appearance of the primitive streak are considered to be simply stages in development of the same embryo. It is assumed, but not proven, that the one and the same embryo continues to exist throughout all stages of development. In other words it is assumed that the zygote continues to exist as the same ontological individual throughout all stages of development. No doubt this stance was taken on account of the obvious continuity of the genetic identity or individuality of the developing embryo. This is quite understandable since no philosophical arguments were given to the Committee to make it think otherwise. Although there are good philosophical reasons to doubt this assumption the Committee felt compelled to advise the Senate that:

> ... it was not persuaded of the inherent ethical validity of the marker event authoritatively put forward in Australia, i.e. the time of the implantation process ... The Committee could see

nothing which marked it as other than a significant event in a continuum of development until birth.[31]

We have already seen (see above, p. 7) that the Committee did allow for the possibility that some marker event might be found before which one could argue beyond reasonable doubt that the human embryo is not yet a true human individual or personal being. As in the case of the Warnock and Waller Committees, the terms of reference of the Australian Senate Select Committee did not include any mention of the timing of when a human individual begins. In the circumstances in which this Senate Committee found itself, and in the absence of any convincing evidence to the contrary, it quite rightly, in my view, argued that the benefit of any reasonable doubt should ethically be resolved in favour of the human embryo.

5   Relevance of natural pregnancy losses

It is sometimes argued, or at least implied, that so many human embryos die before or after implantation that it would be lacking in realism to accept that the human individual begins before implantation. This is so because we would then have to admit that a high proportion of human beings are not even born and never see the light of day ... It is thought this is too hard to accept, especially if one believes in God as a wise and provident Creator. This claim merits some consideration and clarification.

Patricia Jacobs reports that there is evidence that pregnancy losses are high in humans prior to the time when pregnancy is clinically recognized.[32] Up to 50% of ovulated eggs and zygotes recovered after operations were found to be so grossly abnormal that it would be very unlikely that they would result in viable pregnancies. She also suggests that 30% of conceptions detected by positive reactions to human chorionic gonado-trophin (HCG) tests abort spontaneously before these pregnancies are clinically verified. The scientific literature is not unanimous on the incidence of natural wastage prior to, and during, implantation in humans, varying from 15% to as much as 50%.[33] The vast majority of these losses are due to chromosomal defects caused during gametogenesis and fertilization.

It might be consoling to think that these are not yet human persons whose lives are lost. It cannot be argued conclusively, however, from such losses alone, that they could not be human persons on the grounds that it would be contrary to Divine Providence for so many persons to die before reaching the age of reason. For most of human history the infant mortality rate was as high as 50%.[34] In any case, some authorities confidently say up to 25% of clinically recognized pregnancies spontaneously abort.[35] I do not think one can reasonably conclude from this that human embryos several weeks old and fetuses could not be human persons on the grounds that this would conflict with the wisdom of Divine Providence It would indeed be presumptuous to hold that God could not save those who died before the age of reason. We cannot limit God's power, goodness and wisdom as though He were unable to provide eternal happiness for these human individuals who die before being born.

6   Conclusion

The search for an answer to the question of when a human person begins has taken us on a winding and arduous journey of discovery along the inter-connecting pathways of history, philosophy and science. Though the answer is ultimately to be given by philosophical reflection, it has not been easy to determine where to draw the fine line between the competence of science and metaphysics in this delicate exercise of philosophical induction. To a large extent the drawing of this line depends on one's fundamental philosophical outlook. Those who do not favour a metaphysical approach to reality in general tend to draw the line at the stage of development when the emergence of rationally self-conscious acts enables us to relate to such a human individual in a personal way. Some draw the line at the stage of viability when the fetus can survive after birth. Those who give more importance to a metaphysical approach to reality tend to draw the line much earlier in human development. Of these, some are satisfied that a human person is present once a human zygote is constituted with the potential to develop into one or more adult human individuals. Others, myself included, draw the line two weeks later when a living individual human body is actually formed with the active potential to develop further without change in ontological identity.

Instead of viewing development in the first two weeks after fertilization as *development of* the human individual, I have argued the process ought to be regarded as one of *synthesis of* a human individual. We have seen that for about 14 days after fertilization, until the appearance of the primitive streak, the multiplying cells are naturally synthesising a human individual. They have been aptly described as *personne en devenir*.[36] The power of this incipient microscopic human individual to develop and grow from a tiny beginning to adulthood is paralleled by the adult person's ability to trace back one's personal history to that same beginning. A human individual and one's personal history begin together when a living ontological individual with a truly human nature commences development while ever remaining the same individual being.

Though I believe my arguments show that the human individual begins with the appearance of the primitive streak, and not before, it would be presumptuous to declare that my claim was definitely right and opposing opinions were definitely wrong. I have offered my philosophical reflections and reasonings on the scientific evidence now available as a contribution for the search after truth. Even if my arguments are faulty or erroneous, it is necessary to air them so that the truth may eventually emerge. I am sure the debate is far from over. Hopefully the truth will soon appear to the satisfaction of all.

If the thesis I have defended does emerge as the truth, I would suggest that the term 'embryo' be applied from the primitive streak onwards. Prior to this I would suggest that the developing embryonic cells be referred to as 'proembryo' rather than 'pre-embryo' to indicate that though they have not yet become an embryonic human individual they are definitely developing towards that goal.[37] This would avoid the confusion caused by using 'embryo' and 'definitive embryo' and 'embryo proper', as I have done throughout this book following present usage. Logic would favour dissociating 'conception' from 'fertilization' at least when 'conceive' is used by a person in the passive voice. There are good reasons for reserving the active voice of 'conceive' to refer to the completion of implantation as well. This latter change might be more difficult to bring about for the historical and cultural reasons we have already seen. The original meaning of conception has always referred to the beginning of a new life, if not the beginning of the individual eutherian mammal or human person. The biological sciences and technology, it would appear, are not only leaving the law behind, but our culturally entrenched use of terms referring to the beginnings of life and human individuals as well. Hopefully, civilized peoples will be able to respond to the new challenges of our times – not only legal and linguistic, but also ethical as well.

APPENDIXES
Timetable of human prenatal development up to the end of week 10

Caption for Appendixes I, II, III
Development of an ovarian follicle containing an oocyte, ovulation, and the phases of the menstral cycle are illustrated. Development begins at fertilization, about 14 days after the onset of the last menstruation. Cleavage of the zygote in the uterine tube, implantation of the blastocyst, and early development of the embryo are also shown. The main features of developmental stages in human embryos are illustrated. (From K. Moore, *The Developing Human: Clinically Oriented Embryology*. Philadelphia: W. B. Saunders, 3rd edn, 1982, with slight modifications from colour to black and white.)

Appendix I. Timetable of human prenatal development up to the end of week 2.

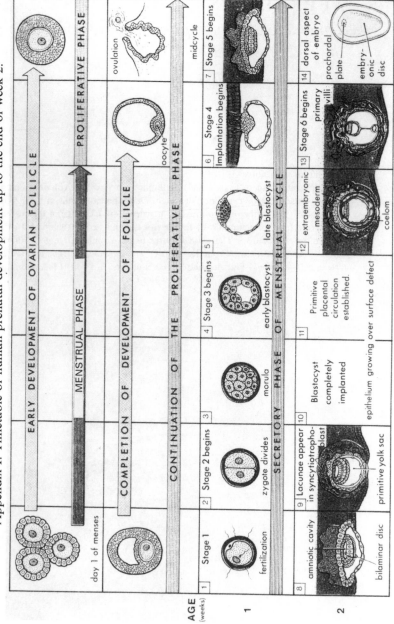

Appendix II. Timetable of human prenatal development: weeks 3 to 6.

15 first missed menstrual period	16 Stage 7 begins	17 intra-embryonic mesoderm	18 Stage 8 begins	19 neural fold	20 Stage 9 begins	21 neural groove
primitive streak	notochordal process	trilaminar embryo	neural plate, primitive streak, length: 1.5 mm	notochord, embryonic coelom	brain, neural groove, somite. Thyroid begins to develop.	somite. Heart tubes begin to fuse.

22 Stage 10 begins	23 rostral neuropore	24 Stage 11 begins	25	26 Stage 12 begins	27	28 Stage 13 begins
Heart begins to beat. Neural folds fusing.	primordia of eye and ear present. caudal neuropore	heart bulge, rostral neuropore closes. 2 pairs of branchial arches	otic pit. 3 pairs of branchial arches	arm bud. indicates actual size	4 pairs of branchial arches, arm & leg buds present. C R = crown-rump length.	C R: 4.0 mm

29	30	31	32	33 Stage 15 begins	34	35
C R: 5.0 mm	Lens pits, optic cups, nasal pits forming.	developing eye, nasal pit, primitive mouth. Lens pits, optic cups and nasal pits forming.	Stage 14. Hand plates (paddle-shaped) Lens pits and optic cups formed.	hand plate. C R: 7.0 mm	Head much larger relative to trunk. cerebral vesicles distinct. leg buds (paddle-shaped)	C R: 8.0 mm

36	37 Stage 16 begins	38	39	40	41 Stage 17 begins	42
Oral & nasal cavities confluent.	foot plate. C R: 9.0 mm	Upper lip formed.	C R: 10.0 mm	Arms bent at elbow. Finger rays and auricular hillocks distinct. Palate developing.	finger rays. ventral view	C R: 13.0 mm

C R = crown-rump length.

3 4 5 6

Appendix III. Timetable of human prenatal development weeks: 7 to 10.

AGE (weeks)

7

43 — CR: 16.0 mm.

44 — Stage 18 begins

45 — Tip of nose distinct / Toe rays appear / Ossification may begin / CR: 17.0 mm

46 — Loss of villi / Smooth chorion forms.

47 — genital tubercle / urogenital membrane / anal membrane / ♀ or ♂

48 — Stage 19 begins / Trunk elongating and straightening

49 — CR: 18 mm

8

50 — Upper limbs longer & bent at elbows / Fingers distinct

51 — Eyelids beginning / Anal membrane perforated / Urogenital membrane degenerating. / Testes and ovaries distinguishable.

52 — Stage 21 begins

53 — Stage 21 / External genitalia still in sexless state but have begun to differentiate.

54 — Stage 22 begins / genital tubercle / urethral groove / anus / ♀ or ♂

55 — Beginnings of all essential external & and internal structures are present.

56 — Stage 23 / CR: 30 mm

9

57 — beginning of fetal period

58 —

59 — Genitalia show some ♀ characteristics but still easily confused with ♂.

60 — phallus / urogenital fold / labioscrotal fold / perineum ♀

61 — Genitalia show fusion of urethral folds. Urethral groove extends into phallus.

62 — phallus / urogenital fold / labioscrotal fold / perineum ♂

63 — CR: 50 mm

10

64 — Face has human profile. Note growth of chin compared to day 44.

65 —

66 — Face has human appearance.

67 — clitoris / labium minus / urogenital groove / labium majus ♀

68 — Genitalia have ♀ or ♂ characteristics but still not fully formed.

69 — glans penis / urethral groove / scrotum ♂

70 — CR: 61 mm

NOTES

Chapter 1

1. *Report of the Committee of Inquiry into Human Fertilisation and Embryology*, Chairman, Dame Mary Warnock, Dept. of Health and Social Security, London: Her Majesty's Stationery Office, 1984, p. 60, 11.15.
2. *Ibid.* p. 90.
3. *Ibid.* p. 63, 11.17.
4. *The Committee to Consider the Social, Ethical and Legal Issues Arising from In Vitro Fertilization: Report on the Disposition of Embryos Produced by In Vitro Fertilization*, Victoria, August 1984, p. 27, 2.8. Cf. also 2.18.
5. *Ibid.* p. 46, 3.27.
6. *Human Embryo Experimentation in Australia: Senate Select Committee on the Human Embryo Experimentation Bill 1985*, Australian Government Publishing Service, Canberra, 1986, pp. 29–30, 3.23.
7. *Ibid.* p. 25, 3.5.
8. *Ibid.* p. 28, 3.18.
9. *Ibid.* p. 28, 3.19.
10. *Ibid.* p. 35, 3.41.
11. *The Oxford English Dictionary*, Oxford: Clarendon Press, 1933, repr. 1961 *s.v.*
12. C. T. Lewis and C. Short, *A Latin Dictionary*, Oxford: Clarendon Press, 1958 *s.v.*
13. *Ibid. s.v.*
14. H. S. Liddell and R. Scott, *A Greek–English Lexicon*, New Ed. revised by Sir H. S. Jones, Oxford: Clarendon Press, 9th edn, 1966. *s.v.*
15. *Ibid. s.v.*
16. *Ibid. s.v.*
17. F. Brown, S. R. Driver, and C. A. Briggs, *A Hebrew and English Lexicon of the Old Testament*, Oxford: Clarendon Press, 1966, *s.v.* p. 247.
18. *Ibid. s.v.*
19. *A Daily Use English-Chinese Dictionary*, Hong Kong: The World Book Company, 1980.
20. Kaizuka, Shigeki *et al.* (ed) *Kadokawa Kanwa Chuujiten*, Tokyo: Kadokawa Shoten, 1973.
21. *Ibid.*
22. Cf. *Usual Vietnamese–English Dictionary*, Nguyen Van Khon, Saigon: Khai Tri. p. 521.

23. *Ibid.* p. 831.
24. *Ibid.* p. 879.
25. Cf. *The Oxford English Dictionary, op. cit. s.v.*
26. Cf. Liddell and Scott, *A Greek–English Lexicon, op. cit. s.v.*
27. Cf. *Ibid. s.v.*
28. Cf. N. M. Ford, S.D.B., 'P. F. Strawson's concept of philosophy', in *Salesianum*, **34** (1972) n. 3, pp. 532–3.
29. For example, human sperm may remain fertile days after the death of the human individual. After death a live heart or kidney may be removed for transplantation for the benefit of another patient.
30. Cf. R. A. Paoletti, 'Developmental-genetic and psycho-social positions regarding the ontological status of the fetus' in *The Linacre Quarterly*, **44**, August, 1977, pp. 250–2.

Chapter 2

1. For a fuller account of Aristotle's embryology and philosophical concepts see Peck's Preface and Introduction to Aristotle, *Generation of Animals*, translated by A. L. Peck, London: W. Heinemann, and Cambridge, Mass.: Harvard University Press, 1963. Cf. also J. Needham, *A History of Embryology*, Cambridge University Press, 1959, esp. pp. 37–60. See pp. 29–37 for Aristotle's resemblance to the views of Empedocles and Hipprocrates. Helpful explanations of Aristotle's theories can also be found *passim* in M. A. Hewson's *Giles of Rome and the Medieval Theory of Conception*, University of London, Athlone Press, 1975.
2. Cf. *The Works of Aristotle*, tr. A. Platt in *The Works of Aristotle Translated into English*, ed. W. D. Ross, Vol. VIII, *Metaphysica*, Oxford: Clarendon Press, 1966, p. 983a: '... causes are spoken of in four senses. In one of these we mean the substance, i.e. the essence (for the 'why' is reducible finally to the definition, and the ultimate 'why' is a cause and principle); in another the matter or substratum, in a third the source of the change and in a fourth the cause opposed to this, the purpose and the good (for this is the end of all generation and change).'
3. *Ibid* 1045b.
4. Cf. *Ibid Metaphysica*, p. 1044a–1044b; Cf. also A. L. Peck, *op. cit.* Introduction, pp. xxxviii–xl.
5. *De Generatione Animalium*, tr. A. Platt in *The Works of Aristotle Translated into English*, Vol. 5, eds. J. A. Smith and W. D. Ross, Oxford: Clarendon Press, 1912, p. 729a. Hereafter referred to as *G.A.* since the Latin title means 'On the Generation of Animals'. All page references to the works of Aristotle are based on Bekker's Greek text. I shall quote A. Platt's translation. Cf. *G.A.* 739a for his general description of conception. Cf. also H. D. Jocelyn and G. P. Setchell, *Regnier De Graaf: On the Human Reproductive Organs* in *Journal of Reproduction and Fertility*, Supp. No. 17, Blackwell Scientific Publications, Oxford, 1972, pp. 136–7, where De Graaf summarizes ten unconvincing reasons why the Aristotelians believe that women do not produce semen (seed) thereby denying them a truly active contribution to the reproductive process.
6. Cf. *G. A.* 729b, where Aristotle shows that he believes the semen does not make any bodily contribution to generation but only the power '... which acts and makes, while that which is made and receives the form is the residue of the secretion in the female'. B. F. Musallam shows how the Muslim religious

thinkers, though following Aristotle to a large extent, depart from him on this point. They follow Hippocrates and Galen who maintained that male and female both contribute equally in fashioning the embryo since both have semen. Cf. *Sex and Society in Islam: Birth Control before the Nineteenth Century*, Cambridge University Press, 1983, Ch. 3 'Conception theory in Muslim thought', pp. 39–59.

7. *G.A.* 729b. The Greeks prized the formal cause far more than the material cause. It is the form that makes a material thing be what it is. Pieces of wood are just that, but once an agent puts them into the form of a chair we speak of a *chair* or wooden *chair* not just pieces *of wood* or *chairish wood*. In their view 'the first efficient or moving cause, to which belongs the definition and the form, is better and more divine in its nature than the material on which it works ... For the first principle of the movement, or efficient cause, whereby that which comes into being is male, is better and more divine than the material whereby it is female'. Cf. *G.A.* 732a. It appears that Aristotle's biological knowledge in this regard to woman's active contribution to human generation was as erroneous as was his mentality chauvinistic!

8. *G.A.* 730a.

9. *G.A.* 730b.

10. Cf. *G.A.* 729a; 737a; 738b; 740b; 743a. Cf. also *G.A.* 736b: 'All have in their semen that which causes it to be productive; I mean what is called vital heat. This is not fire nor any such force, but it is the spiritus [= *pneuma*] included in the semen and the foam-like, and the natural principle in the spiritus, being analogous to the element of the stars.' Here *pneuma*, the bearer of soul, is compared to the *divine* in the heavenly bodies. Little wonder *pneuma* has the power to engender life. Cf. also *G.A.*, 762a: 'Animals and plants come into being in earth and in liquid because there is water in earth, and air in water, and in all air is vital heat, so that in a sense all things are full of soul. Therefore living things form quickly whenever this air and vital heat are enclosed in anything.' I usually use *pneuma* instead of 'air' or 'spiritus' to help the reader bear in mind Aristotle's unique meaning of this term. Think of *pneumatic* tyres filled with air.

11. *G.A.* 728b and *passim*. A. L. Peck's translation is 'fetation', *op. cit.* Cf. his Introduction to *G.A.* paragraph 56 for further comment on its meaning in Aristotle. 'Fetation' possibly refers more to the formation process of the embryo than to the embryo that is formed.

12. Cf. *G.A.* 729a; 737a; 739a and especially 739b: 'When the material secreted by the female in the uterus has been fixed by the semen of the male (this acts in the same way as rennet acts on milk, for rennet is a kind of milk containing vital heat, which brings into one mass and fixes the similar material, and the relation of the semen to the catamenia is the same, milk and the catamenia being of the same nature) – when, I say, the more solid part comes together, the liquid is separated off from it, and as the earthy parts solidify membranes form all round it;' Cf. G.A. 731a: '... the semen forms the embryo in several days.' Cf. also *G.A.* 739b: 'When the embryo is once formed, it acts like the seeds of plants.'

13. Cf. *G.A.* 740b, where Aristotle concedes that the embryo would contain some nourishment for itself, left over from its constitution at the outset. This occurs in plant seeds until they can draw nourishment from the soil through their roots. Aristotle admits this would also be required in the embryo for it to obtain nourishment for its activities prior to the functioning of the blood

circulation system.

14. *The Works of Aristotle Translated in English*, Vol. IV, *The History of Animals* (hereinafter abbreviated as *H.A.*), eds. J. A. Smith and W. D. Ross and translated by D. W. Thompson, Oxford: O.U.P., 1967, p. 583a. Cf. Note 12 above where reference is made to Aristotle's idea that the fluid portion is lost after the bulky portion of the menstrual blood sets. No doubt the 'holding' or 'seizing' on the part of the woman would correspond to what we understand by implantation. Conception is thus presented to be an activity of the woman clinging to what has been formed within her, namely the embryo.

15. *H.A.* 583b.

16. Cf. *G.A.* 729a and 771b–772b. Generally speaking a lack of knowledge of the cell theory, ova and sperm coupled with the potter and clay model of the efficient cause prevented Aristotle even asking himself the question whether what was conceived and formed was a single living individual or many. In this instance he did not adopt the model of efficient cause drawn from the activity of a carpenter who constructs a single house from many separate pieces of wood.

17. *H.A.*, 583b.

18. I am indebted to Dr Marie Dziadek for this suggestion (personal communication).

19. *G.A.* 734a.

20. Cf. *G.A.* 734a, where Aristotle insists on the necessity of contact. Cf. also G.A. 734b, where he explains that a body is in potency to movement until as a result of contact from another body or force it actually begins to move.

21. Cf. *G.A.* 762a. Aristotle's theory applies also to the instances of spontaneous generation that were generally admitted right up to the times of Pasteur. The material that was the equivalent to the female's menstrual blood was earth, sea-water, manure or putrefying flesh, suitably prepared by heat, e.g. the heat of the seasons. *Pneuma* is found in water so it would also be found in fluids or earth's moisture. *Pneuma* is always the instrument of soul, the ultimate life-giving principle. In such cases of asexual spontaneous generation Aristotle was logically forced to admit some specific potentiality was present in the material to account for the different kinds of living beings that originated, in the absence of formal causes comparable to the *pneuma* in the semen of animals. This was necessary because the season's heat and the earth's *pneuma* would be common for all the living creatures produced. Where he could not observe a live bearer of *pneuma* as the instrument of soul, he postulated it to be coherent with his philosophical theory of causes. Cf. Peck's translation of *G.A.*, Appendix B, *op. cit.* pp. 583–6 for more details and references.

22. Cf. Note 6 above and *G.A.* Cf. also *G.A.* 735a, where Aristotle emphasizes that the external movement of nature is taken up from the male parent within the new embryo. Though growth may be dependent on an internal principle, continued development until formation of the being is complete requires a continuing causal input from outside. Cf. *G.A.* 735a: 'Accordingly it is not any part that is the cause of the soul's coming into being, but it is the first moving cause from outside. (For nothing generates itself, though when it has come into being it thenceforward increases itself.)' Cf. also *G.A.* 740b–741a.

23. Cf. *G.A.* 743a: 'But it is not anything whatever that is made into flesh or bone by the heat, but only something naturally fitted for the purpose; nor is it made in any place or time whatever, but only in a place and time naturally so fitted.'

For neither will that which exists potentially be made except by that moving agent which possess the actuality, nor will that which possess the actuality make anything out of anything whatever;'.

24. Cf. *G.A.* 739b.
25. Cf. *G.A.* 740a and G.A. 735a.
26. *G.A.* 744b. Cf. also Aristotle, *On the Soul (De Anima)*, tr. W. S. Hett, London and Cambridge, Mass.: W. Heinemann, 1957, 416b: 'But nutrivity and promotion of growth are not the same; for it is *qua* quantitative that that which has soul has its growth promoted by food, and *qua* individual and substance that it is nourished by it; for it preserves its substance and continues to exist, so long as it is nourished, and it causes the generation not of that which is nourished, but of another like it; for its actual substance already exists, and a thing cannot generate but only preserves itself.'
27. *G.A.* 735a. Cf. also *On the Soul, op. cit.* 415a: '... the nutritive soul belongs to all other living creatures besides man, and is the first most widely shared faculty of the soul, in virtue of which they all have life.'
28. *G.A.* 736b. Aristotle must be referring to the menstrual blood. It is interesting to note he is close to postulating an egg in the female mammal by his line of reasoning.
29. *G.A.* 736b.
30. *On the Soul, op. cit.*, 434a.
31. *Ibid.* 435a. On the same page he also says: 'Without touch there can be no other sense.' But Cf. 415a: 'Touch may exist without any others.' Again Cf. *ibid.* 413b: '... the first characteristic of an animal is sensation ... The first essential factor of sensation, which we all share is a sense of touch. Just as the merely nutritive faculty may exist apart from touch and from all sensation, so touch may exist apart from all other senses.'
32. Cf. *G.A.* 740a.
33. *G.A.* 778b.
34. *G.A.* 731a.
35. Though Aristotle did not define a time for the actual beginning of a human being, and though he was not opposed to abortion for the sake of population control in the state, he was adamant that abortions be performed before sensation and life began in the conceptus. This could indicate that he was aware that the rational soul might be present any time after it was possible to experience sensations, i.e. sometime after 40 days. He makes this point in *Politics*, 1335b: '... there must be a limit fixed to the procreation of offspring, and if any people have a child as a result of intercourse in contravention of these regulations, abortion must be practised on it before it has developed sensation and life; for the line between lawful and unlawful abortion will be marked by the fact of having sensation and being alive'. Cf. Aristotle's *Politics*, tr. H. Rackham, Cambridge, Mass. and Harvard: W. Heinemann, 1967. Cf. also *H.A.* 583b, quoted above (Note 15) where he says most abortions occur before the fortieth day.
36. *G.A.* 736b.
37. Cf. *G.A.*, 740b: 'The real cause why each of them comes into being is that the secretion of the female is potentially such as the animal is naturally, and all the parts are potentially present in it but none actually.' This is only *passive* potency.
38. *G.A.* 741b. 'Air' here refers to the *pneuma* of the father who generates the offspring. The male is needed to give origin to the sensitive soul of the living

animal, as Aristotle says: 'While the body is from the female, it is the soul that is from the male, for the soul is the reality of a particular body.' (*G.A.* 738b) Obviously these views could be used to rationalize male chauvinistic attitudes. By the same token male chauvinistic views could have misled Aristotle in his interpretation of the nature of the female contribution to generation. I am inclined to agree with this latter position, especially in view of his opinions on the nature of the material cause in the case of spontaneous generation (Cf. Note 21 above). Aristotle's erroneous views concerning the woman's contribution to human procreation would have had negative social, cultural and religious repercussions for women for many centuries in Western civilization.

39. *G.A.* 740b. The vital power of *pneuma* may be found in the adult, the embryo, the semen or water. Aristotle is obviously here referring to the vital power of the *pneuma* in the semen derived from the male.

40. Cf. *G.A.* 734a–735b where Aristotle explicitly and in detail argues in favour of epigenesis. He would be logically committed to admit that there must be something in the genetic structure of the embryo to account for the predetermination of the future development of the embryo in an orderly fashion. Today we know of chromosomes and genes, whereas he was left puzzled as to how the homogeneous mass of blood could be predetermined to follow specific developmental pathways when subjected to the causal influence of the semen's *pneuma*. Human *pneuma* could only make a human organism from human blood, not from a cow's blood. He knew the potential would have to be different in each type of blood. There is no questioning that for Aristotle the seed and *pneuma* had to be specific: '... propagation implies a creative seed endowed with certain formative properties.' Cf. *De Partibus Animalium*, tr. W. Ogle in *The Works of Aristotle Translated into English*, eds. J. A. Smith and W. D. Ross, Oxford: Clarendon Press, 1912, 640b. Hereafter referred to as *P.A.* The Latin title means 'Parts of Animals'.

41. Cf. *P.A.* 641b, where Aristotle explains what he means by the purpose or end of a movement. I believe he means a natural movement though he does not explicitly put it this way: 'Again, whenever there is plainly some final end, to which a motion tends should nothing stand in its way, we always say such final end is the aim or purpose of the motion; and from this it is evident that there must be something or other really existing, corresponding to what we call by the name of Nature.' I think this illustrates his meaning of *final cause* in the context of generation.

42. Cf. *P.A.* 641b: 'For a given germ does not give rise to any chance living being, nor spring from any chance one; but each germ springs from a definite parent and gives rise to a definite progeny. And thus it is the germ that is the ruling influence and fabricator of the offspring. For these it is by nature, the offspring being at any rate that which in nature will spring from it. At the same time the offspring is anterior to the germ; for germ and perfected progeny are related as the developmental process and the result.' Cf. also *G.A.* 731a and 739b.

43. *G.A.* 778b. Cf. also *P.A.* 640a: 'For the process of evolution is for the sake of the thing finally evolved, and not this for the sake of the process.' Of course 'evolution' in this context refers to 'formation' or 'development' of the individual, not of the species.

44. *P.A.* 640b.

45. *On the Soul, op. cit.* 416a; Cf. also *G.A.*, 771b–72b and Note 16 above.

46. Cf. *P.A.* 641a: '... it is the presence of the soul that enables matter to constitute the animal nature, much more than it is the presence of matter which so enables the soul...'.

47. *On the Soul, op. cit.* 412b. Cf. also this text a few lines earlier, 412b: 'The soul may therefore be defined as the first actuality of a natural body potentially possessing life; and such will be any body which possesses organs.' Here he means a being is alive if its potential for further life is still being actuated. Death marks the cessation of the actualizing of the potential for organic self-movement.

48. Cf. *On the Soul, op. cit* 412a: 'The soul, then, is the actuality of the kind of body we have described. But actuality has two senses, analogous to the possession of knowledge and the exercise of it. Clearly actuality in our present sense is analogous to the possession of knowledge; for both sleep and waking depend upon the presence of soul, and waking is analogous to the exercising of knowledge, sleep to its possession but not its exercise.'

49. *Ibid.* 415b. Cf. also on the same page: '... for it (soul) is the cause in the sense of being that from which the motion is derived, in the sense of purpose or final cause and as being the substance of all bodies that have souls ... for substance is the cause of existence in all things, and for living creatures existence is life, and of these, the soul is the cause and first principle'.

50. *Ibid.* 415b.

51. Cf. *In III Sententiarum*, Dist. III, Quaest. V., Art. II. The full original text reads as follows:

'Oportet ergo ut conceptio in Christo non praecedat tempore completam naturam carnis eius. Et ita relinquitur quod simul concipiebatur et concepta est.

Propter quod oportet conceptionem illam subitaneam ponere, ita quod haec in eodem instanti fuerint, scilicet **conversio** *sanguinis illius materialis in carnem et alias partes corporis Christi et formatio membrorum organicorum et* **animatio** *corporis organici et* **assumptio** *corporis animati in unitatem divinae personae.*

In aliis autem haec successive contingunt, ita quod maris conceptio non perficitur nisi usque ad quadragesimum diem, ut Philosophus in IX **De Animalibus (De histor. animal.** 3.583b, 2–5) *dicit; feminae autem usque ad nonagesimum. Sed in completione corporis masculi Augustinus videtur superaddere sex dies...'*

It was thought all this time would be taken up with the changing of the blood into flesh, the formation of organs and finally the ensoulment of the organic body to be a man. Augustine thought another six days were needed to total 46! Noonan thinks Augustine and Jerome were not sure about when ensoulment actually occurred. Cf. *The Morality of Abortion: Legal and Historical Perspectives* ed. John T. Noonan Jr, Harvard, Mass: Harvard University Press, 1970, p. 15.

52. *Summa Theologiae*, Ia. 118, I ad 4, *The World Order*, Vol. 15, London: Eyre and Spottiswoode, McGraw-Hill, New York, 1970, ed. and tr. M. J. Charlesworth, pp. 149–51. Cf. also *S. T.* Ia. 76, 3 ad 3; Ia. 92, I; Ia. 115, 2 ad 3 and finally IIIa. 31,5 where the point is made that the female material i.e. the blood, is specially prepared by the mother to be '*materia apta ad conceptum*' i.e. 'suitable matter for conception'. Cf. also J. Needham, *op. cit.* pp. 22, 92–3 and 236 for some enlightening comments on Aquinas' and others' *theological embryology* as opposed to scientific embryology. Cf. also M. A. Hewson, *op. cit. passim*, for references to Aquinas' thoughts on human reproduction. Cf. also *Summa Contra Gentiles*, II, Ch. 86–9.

53. *S. T.* Ia. 118, 2 ad 2, *op. cit.* p. 153.

54. *Ibid.* p. 155. Aquinas here re-echoes what Aristotle had previously said: 'The facts regarding the soul are much the same as those relating to figures; for both

in figures and in things which possess soul, the earlier type always exists
potentially in that which follows; e.g. the triangle is implied in the quadri-
lateral, and the nutritive faculty by the sensitive.' Cf. *On the Soul, op. cit.* 415a.
Cf. also *De Spiritualibus Creaturis*, Art. 3c ad 13. Cf. also *S.T.* II–IIae, 64, 8 ad
2, where Aquinas holds that one would be guilty of homicide if the death either
of the mother or of the ensouled fetus were to result from a blow to a pregnant
woman. No doubt Aquinas would have been well aware of, and approved, the
quotation of the fifth-century theologian Gennadius of Marseilles, included by
Peter Lombard in his *Book of Sentences*: 'We affirm that only the Creator of all
knows the creation of the soul; that in intercourse only the body is sown, which
by God's decree becomes coagulated inside the womb, and is developed and
formed; and that once the body has been formed the soul is created and poured
in, so that in the womb there is a living man consisting of soul and body, and
what emerges alive from the womb is a man complete in human substance.'
Quoted in *Bioethics and Belief*, by John Mahoney, Sheed and Ward, London,
1984, p. 72.

55. *S.T.*, Ia. 76, 4, ad 1 *op. cit.* Vol. 11, ed. and tr. T. Suttor, p. 69. In *De
Spiritualibus Creaturis*, Art. 3c, he stresses that the form is act and consequently is the reason for the unity in a being. This is why there can be only one
substantial form in an individual being. Cf. also *ibid.* art. 4c, where Aquinas
points out that the soul needs different organs in different parts of the body.
The more perfect the soul, the greater the differention needed for its activities
within the unity of the whole organism. Cf. also *Summa Contra Gentiles* II,
Ch. 89 *passim*.

56. Cf. *S. T.* IIIa. 33, 1c. After speaking of the formation of the body of Christ
from the blood he refers to '... *ipsa formatio corporis in qua principaliter ratio
conceptionis consistit ...*'. My translation would be: '... the formation itself of
the body wherein the notion of conception principally consists ...'. There is an
active and passive side to this formation. The active power of the *pneuma* in the
semen shapes or forms, while the embryo itself is formed from within. Of
course, a human being only exists when the requisite formation is completed.
In *S.T.* IIIa, 6, 4 ad 1, referring to the case of Christ he states '*ante adventum
animae non est caro humana*', i.e. that there is no true human flesh before
rational ensoulment. Yet in his reply to the next objection he says: 'caro nostra
prius concipitur quam animetur', i.e. that *our* flesh is conceived before it is
ensouled. Notice he says the flesh is conceived, not the human being in *our*
case. We should not forget that Aquinas at times uses the term *conceive* to refer
to the complete process and at other times to the start only, before rational
ensoulment.

57. Aquinas was conditioned by the conventional use of the term in his times. He
could not make a clean break with the Aristotelian meaning of *conceive*, except
in the case of Christ. Little wonder, as this was a miraculous conception and a
mystery beyond human comprehension in any case. When Aquinas came to
discuss the Immaculate Conception of the Virgin Mary in the context of all
men being redeemed by the saving grace of Christ, he realized she could not
have been sanctified before rational ensoulment occurred for the simple reason
that *she* could not be guilty of original sin if she did not yet exist as a personal
being with a rational soul. Cf. *S.T.*, IIIa, 27, 2: '*ante infusionem animae
rationalis proles concepta non est culpae obnoxia*'. i.e. 'before the infusion of the
rational soul, the offspring that is conceived is not subject to guilt'. Here he
admits of a conception in the case of Mary, followed in due time by ensoul-

ment and sanctification. The solution of course is that she was sanctified in the first instant of *her* existence (= personal conception in the passive sense) without any reference to the time of this holy conception nor to conception in the active sense. Aquinas could not have recourse to a miraculous and instantaneous conception as he did in the case of Christ 'conceived by the power of the Holy Spirit'. This was unique for Christ as God and man. Cf. also *S.T.* IIIa., 33, 2, where Aquinas discusses the case of Christ more fully. He does admit the size of the body of Christ would have been much smaller than usual, but it still would have been properly formed in proportion to its size at that stage. However, it is true to say that Aquinas was anxious to say that the Virgin Mary was carrying Jesus within her womb from the very beginning of the miraculous conception of Christ. The fruit of her conception by the power of the Holy Spirit was to be from the start both Son of God and son of the Virgin Mother. This Christian dogma of the miraculous conception of Christ (Virgin Birth) cannot shed light on the moment of natural conception or rational ensoulment. Christ's coming into this world is like his leaving of this world: it is quite beyond our experience, understanding and the normal laws of nature because God's infinite and mysterious power is directly involved. For more on the meanings of active and passive conception see *The Dogma of the Immaculate Conception: History and Significance*, ed. Edward O. O'Connor, C.S.C., Notre Dame: University of Notre Dame Press, 1958, pp. 133–4; 147; 173; 332–4; 526.

58. William Harvey, *Disputations Touching the Generation of Animals*, tr. with intro. by Gweneth Whitteridge, Oxford: Blackwell Scientific Publications, 1981, p. 17. Cf. also p. XLIV. Harvey's findings were published in Latin in 1651 and in English in 1653. Cf. William Harvey, *Anatomical Exercitations Concerning the Generation of Living Creatures*, tr. M. Llewellyn, London: Pulleyn, 1653. Also tr. R. Willis, London: Sydenham Society, 1847. Cf. the following useful references to Harvey's works, J. Needham, *op. cit.* pp. 133–53, where Harvey's work and achievements are thoroughly outlined. E. B. Gasking, *Investigations into Generations: 1651–1828*, London: Hutchinson, 1967, pp. 16–36; R. V. Short, 'Harvey's Conception: '*De Generatione animalium*', 1651' in *Developments in Cardiovascular Medicine*, eds. C. J. Dickinson and J. Marks, M.T.P. Press, Lancaster, 1978, pp. 353–63.

59. Harvey, tr. Whitteridge, *op. cit.* p. li, where Harvey's *Anatomical Lectures* of 1616 are quoted.

60. *Ibid.* p. 332.

61. Cf. R. V. Short, 'Harvey's Conception: 'De Generatione animalium', 1651', *art. cit.* pp. 356–60.

62. Harvey, tr. Whitteridge, *op. cit.* pp. 353–4. Exercise 68. *Semen* would be a more accurate translation than *sperm* as *sperm* were not seen until after Harvey's death. In this respect the early translations by Llewellyn and Willis were better. Cf. R. V. Short, 'Harvey's Conception', *art. cit.* pp. 361–2.

63. Harvey, tr. Whitteridge, *op. cit.* p. 344.

64. *Ibid.* p. 444. See comment on translation in Note 62.

65. *Ibid.* p. 448. Cf. also p. 227.

66. *Ibid.* pp. 238–9.

67. *Ibid.* p. 445.

68. *Ibid.* p. 452.

69. Cf. Joseph Needham, *A History of Embryology*, Cambridge University Press, 1959, pp. 119–20 and 257 where he refers to the following: Thomas Fienus

(Feyens, Fyens), *De Formatrice Foetus, in quo ostenditur animam rationalem infundi tertia die,* Antwerp: Tong, 1620. Its translation: '*On the Formation of the Fetus, in Which it is Shown the Rational Soul is Infused on the Third Day*'.

70. Joseph Needham, *op. cit.* p. 120.
71. Cf. also Germain Grisez, *Abortion: the Myths, the Realities and the Arguments,* N.Y.: Corpus Book, The World Publishing Co., 1972, pp. 170–1.
72. Cf. *Ibid.* pp. 171–2. *Cf.* also John T. Noonan, Jr, ed. *The Morality of Abortion– Legal and Historical Perspectives,* Harvard, 1972, pp. 34–6.
73. Cf. Noonan, *op. cit.* p. 35.
74. *Ibid.* p. 35.
75. Short *art. cit.* p. 353. For an account of those who first thought sperm entered eggs from 1843 (Barry) to 1853 (Newport) and who described fertilization from 1875 (Van Benedin), 1876 (Hertwig) to 1895 (Sobotta), see *The Mammalian Egg,* C. R. Austin, Oxford: Blackwell Scientific Publications, 1961, pp. 4–6.
76. J. Needham, *op. cit.* p. 205. Cf. also pp. 121, 206. Cf. E. B. Gasking, *op. cit.* pp. 42–3.
77. E. Anscombe and P. T. Geach (trs. and eds.), *Descartes: Philosophical Writings,* London: Nelson's University Paperbacks, The Open University, repr. 1975, p. 32.
78. Noonan, *op. cit.* p. 38.
79. Cf. J. Donceel, 'Immediate Animation and Delayed Hominization' in *Theological Studies,* **31** (1970) 76–105, esp pp. 91–2.
80. *Ibid.* p. 82.
81. *Ibid.* p. 83. Cf. also Donceel's *Philosophical Anthropology,* New York: Sheed and Ward, 1967, pp. 440–5.
82. Donceel, 'Immediate Animation and Delayed Hominization', *art. cit.* p. 98.
83. *Ibid.* Cf. pp. 98–9.
84. Cf. *Ibid.* pp. 98–9. Cf. also P. Schoonenberg, *God's World in the Making,* Dublin: Gill and Son, 1965, pp. 49–50.
85. Donceel, 'Immediate Animation and Delayed Hominization', *art. cit.* p. 101.
86. Cf. the following: B. Haring, 'New Dimensions of Responsible Parenthood' in *Theological Studies,* **37** (1976) 125–9; *Free and Faithful in Christ,* Vol. 3, Homebush: St. Paul Publication, 1981, pp. 5–10.
    J. J. Diamond, M.D. 'Abortion, Animation and Biological Hominization' in *Theological Studies,* **36** (1975) 305–24. Dr. Diamond provides more biological evidence than most philosophers and theologians. This makes this contribution more valuable. See especially p. 315.
    G. Pastrana, 'Personhood and the Beginning of Human Life' in *The Thomist,* **41** (1977) 247–94. This also contains a good survey of contemporary opinions. See especially pp. 281–2.
    K. Rahner, *Theological Investigations,* Vol. 9, '*Writings 1965–7, I,* Darton, Longman & Todd, London, 1972, pp. 226 and 236.
    P. O'Mahony, 'Where human life begins', in *The Month,* Dec. 1977, pp. 400–5.
87. Cf. Grisez, *op. cit.* pp. 117–35. Cf. also Needham, *op. cit.,* pp. 18–37, esp. for the views of Anaxagoras of Clazomenae (500–428 B.C.) Empedocles (d. 444 B.C.) and the unknown Hippocratic embryologist. It appears some of their views could have indirectly influenced some of the expressions in biblical writings.
88. *The Book of Job* (10: 8–12). The similarities to the doctrines of Aristotle are obvious in this passage. Of course this could very well mean that Aristotle and the author of Job obtained these views from some earlier common sources. Not

all of Aristotle's views are original. He definitely depended on earlier writers and traditions for some of his general conceptions. Job would have been written most likely before the time of Aristotle, possibly about 450 B.C. Other relevant passages are: *Jeremiah* 1: 5; *Psalm* 139: 13–16; *2 Maccabees* 7: 22–3. All quotations are taken from *The Jerusalem Bible*, published and copyright 1966, 1967 and 1968 by Darton, Longman and Todd Ltd and Doubleday & Co. Inc. and are used by permission of the publishers.

89. Cf. Needham, *op. cit.* p. 21.
90. M. Fishbane discusses this text and is inclined to agree, though he admits it is ambiguous. Cf. *Biblical Interpretation in Ancient Israel*, Clarendon Press, Oxford, 1985, pp. 91–4. Cf. also Les Miller, *A Christian View on In Vitro Fertilization*, Sydney: Anglican Information Office, 1985, pp. 32–8. He argues that the text could also be interpreted differently to imply that the early fetus was invested with full human rights. He presents various views. His final word is inconclusive in regard to resolving the dilemma of the moral status of the early human embryo on biblical grounds.
91. Cf. Grisez, *op. cit.* p. 127, where he quotes A. E. Crawley on this point.
92. *The Septuagint with Apocrypha: Greek and English*, tr. Sir Lancelot C. L. Brenton, Grand Rapids, Michigan: Zondervan Publishing House, Tenth Printing 1970, first printed 1851, p. 98. When the medieval canonists thought that abortion, performed before rational ensoulment had occurred, was not the moral equivalent of homicide, they were influenced by the thinking behind the Septuagint translation. Cf. *Corpus Iuris Canonici: Decretum Gratiani*, Vol. I, ed. A. Friedberg, Graz: Akademische Druck-u. Verlagsanstalt, 1959, C. 32. q. 2. cc. 8, 9, 10, pp. 1122.
93. Cf. Grisez, *op. cit.* p. 131, where he correlates this translation to something similar in the Hittite Laws, about 1500 B.C. where the penalty is graded according to the month of pregnancy. This only shows that prior to Aristotle, stages of human fetal development, and consequently of legal sanctions, were gauged in terms of the length of the pregnancy and fetal development. This would be over a thousand years before Aristotle's birth. Cf. also G. R. Dunstan, 'The Moral Status of the Human Embryo: A Tradition Recalled', in *The Journal of Medical Ethics*, **10** (1984) 38–44.
94. Cf. Grisez, *op. cit.* p. 131. Cf. also Noonan, *op. cit.* p. 6.
95. Philo, *The Works of Philo Judaeus, The Contemporary of Josephus*, Vol III, tr. C. D. Yonge, London, Covent Garden: Henry G. Bohn, 1855, p. 330. See also *Philo VII, The Special Laws*, III, 108–9, tr. F. H. Colson, Cambridge, Mass.: Harvard, and London: W. Heinemann, 1968, p. 545 for a modern English version.
96. *Gospel of St. Luke* 1: 41–4.
97. *Declaration on Procured Abortion*, issued by the S. Congregation for the Doctrine of the Faith, 18 Nov. 1974, published in *Vatican Council II: More Postconciliar Documents*, ed. A. Flannery, O. P. Dublin: Dominican Publications, 1982, p. 443. More details on the history of these issues can be found in Noonan, *op. cit.* pp. 9–46 and Grisez *op. cit.* pp. 137–84.
98. Grisez, *op. cit.*, pp. 177. Cf. Noonan, *op. cit.* p. 39.
99. Cf. P. Schoonenberg, *God's World in the Making*, Dublin: Gill and Son, 1965, p. 65. Cf. also *The Dogma of the Immaculate Conception*, ed. E. O'Connor, Notre Dame University Press, 1958, pp. 332–5.
100. *The Teaching of the Catholic Church*, ed. K. Rahner, New York: Alba House, 1967, p. 122. Cf. also Donceel, *art. cit.* pp. 86–8.
101. Vatican II, *Gaudium et Spes*, n. 51. Cf. also my article 'Catholic Teaching in

Relation to In Vitro Fertilization Within Marriage' in *The Australasian Catholic Record*, **60** (1983) Note 13, p. 414 for an account of the earlier draft and significance of this statement. See also my articles 'Human Experimentation' in *The Australasian Catholic Record*, **61** (1984) 75–80; 'Moral Issues that Arise in Experimentation on Human Embryos' in *The Australasian Catholic Record*, **63** (1986), 3–20.

102. *Declaration on Procured Abortion*, Cf. Flannery, *loc. cit.*, pp. 445–6. Cf. also J. Mahoney, *Bioethics and Belief: Religion and Medicine in Dialogue*, London: Sheed and Ward, 1984, pp. 67–83 for a longer discussion of the *Declaration* and related issues. The Church also teaches that it pertains to the competence of doctors to give a precise definition of death and of the moment of death. Pope Pius XII points out that death takes place at the complete and definitive separation of soul and body. However, in practice it is necessary to bear in mind the imprecise notion of the terms 'body' and 'separation'. These matters cannot be deduced from religious or moral principles. Cf. Pius XII in *Acta Apostolicae Sedis*, **49** (1957) 1031, 1033.

103. *Declaration on Procured Abortion*, in Flannery, *op. cit.* p. 452. It is right to say one cannot prove there is no rational soul once a human individual is present.

104. Pope John Paul II, *L'Osservatore Romano*, Weekly Edition in English, N. 49 (966), 9 December 1986, p. 14.

105. *Ibid.* Pope John Paul II, p. 13.

106. Congregation for the Doctrine of the Faith, *Instruction on Respect for Human Life in its Origin and on the Dignity of Procreation – Replies to Certain Questions of the Day*, Vatican City: Vatican Polyglot Press, 1987, p. 6.

107. *Ibid.* p. 13.

108. *Ibid.* p. 3, modified to conform to the official Latin text in *Acta Apostolicae Sedis*, **80** (1988) 71.

109. *Ibid.* p. 13, modified to conform to the Latin text in *ibid.* pp. 78–9. Cf. *Acta Apostolicae Sedis*, **80** (1988) 78–9 for the official Latin text, published during the final proofs of this book, where it says that respect is due 'from the beginning of the formation of the zygote' (p. 78), defined as 'the cell that arises from the fusion of two gametes'. (p. 79) Ch. 4, Note 3 explains why the definition is less specific.

110. *Ibid.* p. 18, modified to conform to the Latin text in *ibid.* p. 83.

Chapter 3

1. Jenny Teichman, 'Wittgenstein on Persons and Human Beings' in *Royal Institute of Philosophy Lectures*, London, Vol. 7, 1972–1973, p. 140.

2. John Locke, *Essay Concerning Human Understanding*, Book II, Ch. 27, para. 9. and 26. Cf also paras. 6–8.

3. P. F. Strawson, *Individuals, An Essay in Descriptive Metaphysics*, London: Methuen, University Paperbacks, 1959, pp. 101–2.

4. P. Singer, *Practical Ethics*, Cambridge University Press, 1979, p. 76.

5. M. Tooley, *Abortion and Infanticide*, Oxford: Clarendon Press, 1983, p. 123. Cf. also pp. 123–34; 146; 303; 419–20.

6. P. Singer and D. Wells, *The Reproductive Revolution: New Ways of Making Babies*, Oxford: Oxford University Press, 1984, p. 90. Cf. also W. Walters and P. Singer in *Test-Tube Babies*, Melbourne: Oxford University Press 1982, p. 60.

7. M. Lockwood, ed., *Moral Dilemmas in Modern Medicine*, Oxford: Oxford University Press, 1985, p. 10.

8. J. Harris, 'In Vitro Fertilization: The Ethical Issues' in *The Philosophical Quarterly*, **33** (1983) No. 132, p. 225.

9. Mary Warnock, '*In Vitro* Fertilisation: The Ethical Issues' (II), *The Philosophical Quarterly*, **33** (1983) No. 132, p. 239.
10. *Ibid.* p. 239–42.
11. Mary Warnock, 'Do Human Cells Have Rights?', *Bioethics*, **1** (1987) 2–3.
12. When death occurs more than one new form could very well emerge to give rise to more than one entity.
13. Cf. A. G. Van Melson, *The Philosophy of Nature*, Pittsburg: Duquesne University Press, 1961, pp. 115–25 for an exposition of the species-individual structure of matter. See also B. van Hagens, *Filosofia della Natura*, Rome: Urbiana University Press, 1983, pp. 157–63, on how it is possible for there to be many individuals of the same type.
14. H. Kuhse and P. Singer, *Should the Baby Live? The Problem of Handicapped Infants*, Oxford: Oxford University Press, 1985, p. 133.
15. Cf. P. Singer, *Practical Ethics*, Cambridge University Press, 1979, pp. 97–8. Cf. also P. Singer and D. Wells, *The Reproduction Revolution: New Ways of Making Babies*, Oxford: Oxford University Press, 1984, pp. 89–98. M. Lockwood, *op. cit.* p. 10.
16. Cf. M. Lockwood, *op. cit.* p. 10.
17. *Ibid.* p. 13.
18. Cf. *Ibid*, p. 19.
19. Cf. *Ibid.* pp. 22–3; Note 18, p. 212.
20. *Ibid.* p. 23. Oliver O'Donovan thinks the functioning brain criterion of personhood represents a *qualitative* concept of person rather than one where the person is viewed as the subject of rational nature, qualities and attributes. I am in agreement with the thrust of his comments when he says the account 'which relates personal identity to brain-function is inconclusive because it rests on a *philosophical* preference rather than a scientific one, a preference for *qualitative* conceptions of personal identity such as the early Christian thinkers confronted and found wanting ... the individual substance ... does not point to a quality, or complex of qualities, but to a "someone who"!' *Begotten or Made?*, Oxford: Clarendon Press, 1984, pp. 57–9.
21. Cf. P. Jacobs, 'Pregnancy Losses and Birth Defects' in *Embryonic and Fetal Development*, Book 2, *Reproduction in Mammals*, eds. C. R. Austin and R. V. Short, Cambridge University Press, 1982, pp. 152–4. The hydatidiform mole was well known to Aristotle as this account shows: 'We must also speak of what is known as *mola uteri*, which occurs rarely in women but still is found sometimes during pregnancy. For they produce what is called a *mola*; it has happened before now to a woman, after she had intercourse with her husband and supposed she had conceived, that at first the size of her belly increased and everything else happened accordingly, but yet when the time for birth came on, she neither bore a child nor was her size reduced, but she continued thus for three or four years until dysentery came on, endangering her life, and she produced a lump of flesh which is called a *mola*. Moreover this condition may continue until old age and death. ... (For their nature seems to be incapable, and unable to perfect or put the last touches to the process of generation. Hence it is that the *mola* remains in them till old age or at any rate for a long time, for in its nature it is neither perfect nor altogether a foreign body.)' Cf. Aristotle, *De Generatione Animalium*, tr. Arthur Platt, in *The Works of Aristotle Translated into English*, eds. J. A. Smith and W. D. Ross, Vol. V, Oxford: Clarendon Press, 1912, pp. 775b–76a.
22. Cf. K. Moore, *The Developing Human: Clinically Oriented Embryology*, 3rd.

ed., Philadelphia: W. B. Saunders, 1982, p. 57. These cells are genetically unique as well. Cf. P. J. O'Mahony and M. Potts, 'Abortion and the Soul' in *The Month*, **38** (1967) 48.

23. *Summa Theologiae (S.T.)* III, Q. 16, art. 12 ad 1, London: Eyre and Spottiswoode, and New York: McGraw-Hill, 1965, vol. 50, ed. C. E. O'Neill, O. P. p. 45. Cf. also S. T. I, Q. 29, 1.

24. *Ibid.* art. 12 ad 2.

25. John Mahoney, S. J. *Bioethics and Belief*, London: Sheed and Ward, 1984, p. 64. Cf. also pp. 64–6. Most likely Mahoney would have been aware of similar views held by Haring, Diamond, Pastrana and Rahner – see Note 86 in Ch. 2 above for references.

26. M. Warnock, '*In Vitro* Fertilization: The Ethical Issues (II)', in *The Philosophical Quarterly*, **33** (1983) No. 132, p. 241. She subsequently expressed similar views in 'Do Human Cells Have Rights?' in *Bioethics*, **1** (1987) 10–11, attributing her views to the majority of the Warnock Committee.

27. *Op. cit.* Aquinas, *S.T.*, I, Q. 29, art. 4. Vol. 6. ed. C. Velechy O.P., p. 59.

28. David Holbrook sounds a warning against attempts made to reduce life to something purely chemical, physical and mechanical. The biological cannot be treated as if it were inorganic, as though the chemical alone was real. Living beings develop and exist in time and have an irreducible meaning. Cf. 'Medical ethics and the potentialities of the living being', in *British Medical Journal*, **291** (1985) 459–62.

29. John Locke supplied the reasons for this in the following words: '… in these two cases – a *mass of matter* and a *living body* – identity is not applied to the same things'. *op. cit.* Ch. 27, para. 3.

30. The growing crystal is not alive. More of the same type of molecules take on the crystalline form to increase the size of an individual crystal (e.g. alum). This is not an immanent action of nutrition or growth, but simply a process of integration and enlargement following the juxtaposition or aggregation of additional molecules. A similar process occurs when atoms interact to form a more complex and larger molecule.

31. John Locke, *op. cit.* Ch. 27, para. 6.

32. E. S. Russell, *The Directiveness of Organic Activities*, Cambridge University Press, 1945, p. 190.

33. In this I differ from the following: P. Singer and D. Wells, *op. cit.* pp. 90–1; W. Walters and P. Singer, *op. cit.* p. 61; M. Warnock, 'Do Human Cells Have Rights?', *Bioethics*, **1** (1987) 12. 'To say that eggs and sperm cannot by themselves become human, but only if bound together, does not seem to me to differentiate them from the early embryo which by itself will not become human either, but will die unless it is implanted. In short, I do not think that the concept of *potentiality* has any precise sense which will necessitate the treatment of early embryos as requiring the full protection of the law.'

34. *Report of the Committee of Inquiry into Human Fertilisation and Embryology*, Chairman Dame Mary Warnock, Dept. of Health and Social Security, London: Her Majesty's Stationery Office, 1984, p. 63, 11.17.

35. *Ibid.* p. 90.

36. Cf. Mary Warnock, '*In Vitro* Fertilization: The Ethical Issues (II)', *art. cit.* p. 241. She spells out her thinking further: 'The question whether or not they (= human embryos) may be used in research must be answered, not with regard to their potentiality, but with regard to what they are … how far they

are along the long road to becoming fully human.' Cf. 'Do Human Cells have Rights?' *art. cit.* p. 12. Of course their proximate potentiality consists precisely in their actual genetically human life and their closeness to becoming truly human individuals.
37. Clifford Grobstein, a biologist, makes the same point: 'Moreover, developmental individuality appears to be pre-requisite to personhood, though the two terms are not equivalent.' Cf. 'The Moral Use of Spare Embryos' in *The Hastings Center Report*, June, 1982, p. 6.

Chapter 4

1. I have drawn from the following sources for information on fertilization:
   K. Moore, *The Developing Human: Clinically Oriented Embryology*, 3rd edn, Philadelphia: W. B. Saunders, 1982, pp. 1–32. Bruce Alberts *et al.*, *Molecular Biology of the Cell*, New York: Garland Publishing, Inc., 1983, pp. 776–809.
   J. M. Bedford, 'Fertilization' in *Germ Cells and Fertilization*, Book I, *Reproduction in Mammals*, eds. C. R. Austin and R. V. Short, Cambridge University Press, 1982, pp. 128–62; A. G. Byskov, 'Primordial germ cells and regulation of meiosis', *ibid.* pp. 1–17; T. G. Baker, 'Oogenesis and ovulation', *ibid.* pp. 17–45.
   L. Mohr and A. Trounson 'In Vitro Fertilization and Embryo Growth' in *Clinical In Vitro Fertilization* eds. C. Wood and A. Trounson, Berlin: Springer-Verlag, 1984, pp. 99–108. A. H. Sathananthan *et al.*, *Atlas of Fine Structure of Human Sperm Penetration, Eggs and Embryos Cultured 'In Vitro'*, New York: Praeger Publishers, 1986, pp. 85–112.
2. Cf. M. J. K. Harper, 'Sperm and Egg Transport' in *Germ Cells and Fertilization*, Book 2, *Reproduction in Mammals*, eds C. R. Austin & R. V. Short, Cambridge University Press, 1982, pp. 109, 111 and 112. It is possible for sperm to survive after coitus in the fallopian tube folds for 2–3 days.
3. Moore, Bedford, Mohr and Trounson all agree on this point of the completion of the process of fertilization. Moore sets the limit for fertilization at 24 hours for humans, cf. p. 30. The earliest stage possible to claim that fertilization results in the formation of a new genetically unique individual is reached when the sperm contents are released into the egg and the second polar body is extruded, whereby the oocyte is left in the haploid state and the maturation of the ovum is completed.
4. Cf. G. J. V. Nossal, *Reshaping Life: Key Issues in Genetic Engineering*, Melbourne and Cambridge: Melbourne University Press, 1984, pp. 13–21. More information on cell structures and functions can be found in standard texts. Cf. *Biological Science: The Web of Life*, Australian Academy of Science, Canberra, 1975, pp. 623–33.
5. R. Edwards and P. Steptoe, *A Matter of Life*, London: Sphere, 1981, p. 91.
6. Cf. R. G. Edwards, 'Test-tube babies: the ethical debate', The Horizon Lecture, in *The Listener*, 27 Oct. 1983, p. 12; J. J. Diamond, M.D., 'Abortion, Animation and Biological Hominization' in *Theological Studies,* **36** (1975) 305–24, esp. p. 315.
7. T. V. Daly, S.J. 'The Status of Embryonic Human Life – A Crucial Issue in Genetic Counselling' in *Health Care Priorities in Australia: Proceedings of the 1985 Annual Conference on Bioethics*, ed. N. Tonti-Filippini, Melbourne: St Vincent's Bioethics Centre, 1985, pp. 52. This article with minor modifications was submitted as evidence to the *Senate Select Committee on The Human Embryo Bill 1985* in *Experimenting With the Origins of Human Lives*, eds. N.

Tonti-Filippini and T. V. Daly, S. J. Melbourne, St Vincent's Bioethics Centre, 1986, pp. 45–59, and published in the *Official Hansard Report* as part of the evidence heard on 25 February 1986 in Melbourne, *Evidence*, pp. 188–9.

8. Cf. C. R. Austin, 'The Egg' in *Germ Cells and Fertilization*, Book 1, *Reproduction in Mammals*, eds. C. R. Austin & R. V. Short, Cambridge University Press, 1982, pp. 53–4; A. McLaren, 'The Embryo' in *Embryonic and Fetal Development*, Book 2, *Reproduction in Mammals*, Cambridge University Press, 1982, pp. 12–4. The four-cell stage is suggested for the expression of the human embryonic genome by P. R. Braude, V. N. Bolton and M. H. Johnson in 'The use of human pre-embryos for research,' in *Human Embryo Research: Yes or No?*, The Ciba Foundation, London: Tavistock Publications, 1986, p. 68. Anne McLaren up-dates her views in this same book in 'Prelude to embryogenesis', *ibid*, pp. 6–9.

9. T. V. Daly *art. cit.* p. 53, and *Hansard op. cit.*, p. 189.

10. *Ibid.* pp. 55 and 191.

11. B. M. Ashley, O.P. 'Pro-Life Evangelization' in *New Technologies of Birth and Death: Medical, Legal and Moral Dimensions*, St Louis, Missouri: Pope John XXIII Medical–Moral Research and Education Centre, 1980, p. 85.

12. T. W. Hilgers, M.D., 'The New Technologies of Birth and Death', *ibid.* p. 34.

13. Quoted in the *Report on the Disposition of Embryos Produced by In Vitro Fertilization, The Committee to Consider the Social, Ethical and Legal Issues Arising from In Vitro Fertilization*, Melbourne, August, 1984, Appendix A, Statement of Dissent by Rev. Dr Francis Harman, p. 64.

14. Cf. B. M. Ashley, O.P., 'A Critique of the Theory of Delayed Animation' in *An Ethical Evaluation of Fetal Experimentation: An Interdisciplinary Study*, eds. D. G. McCarthy and A. S. Moraczewski, O.P., St. Louis, Missouri: Pope John XXIII Medical–Moral Research and Education Center, 1976, App. I, pp.113–33. See also pp. 21–40.
B. M. Ashley, O.P. and K. D. O'Rourke, O.P. *Health Care Ethics: A Theological Analysis*, St Louis: The Catholic Health Association of USA, 1982, pp. 218–27.
W. E. May, *Human Existence, Medicine and Ethics*, Chicago: Franciscan Herald Press, 1977, pp. 93–105.
S. O'Reilly, M.D. *Bioethics and the Limits of Science*, Front Royal, Virginia: Christendom Publications, 1979, pp. 70–84.
T. Iglesias, 'In Vitro Fertilisation: the major issues' in *Journal of Medical Ethics* (1984) **1**, 32–7; *A Basic Ethic for Man's Wellbeing: Conscience and the New Scientific Possibilities*, Merseyside, World Federation of Doctors who Respect Human Life, British Section, 1984, pp. 9–14.

15. K. Moore, *op. cit.* pp. 1 and 14.

16. J. A. F. Roberts, *An Introduction to Medical Genetics*, 3rd edn, Oxford: Oxford University Press, 1963, p. 1.

17. G. Simpson and W. Beck, *Life: An Introduction to Biology*, 2nd edn, London: Harcourt Brace, 1965, p. 139.

18. W. J. Hamilton and H. W. Mossman, *Human Embryology*, Cambridge: Heffer, 4th edn, 1972, p. 14.

19. B. M. Patten, *Human Embryology*, New York: McGraw Hill, 3rd. edn, 1968, p. 43.

20. Cf. G. C. Liggins, 'Fetal Development and Birth' in *Embryonic and Fetal Development*, Book 2, *Reproduction in Mammals*, eds. C. R. Austin & R. V. Short, Cambridge University Press, 1982, p. 118.

21. A similar line of reasoning is adopted by G. E. M. Anscombe in 'Were You a Zygote?' in *Philosophy and Practice*, ed. A. Phillips Griffiths, Cambridge University Press, 1985, pp. 111–15. Cf. also P. T. Geach in *The Virtues*, Cambridge University Press, 1977, p. 30 where he asserts that the fertilized egg is not a human being.

22. *Official Hansard Report* of the *Senate Select Committee on the Human Embryo Experimentation Bill 1985*, Evidence heard in Canberra, 10 March 1986, pp. 1086, 1088.

23. *Ibid.* p. 1102.

24. Report of the U.S. Senate Subcommittee on the Separation of Powers. Evidence given on 23 April 1981, p. 9. There is also a French version of this statement, 'Le debut de l'etre humain', published in *La Revue du Praticien*, tome XXX 1, n. 32, pp. 2327–8.

25. Cf. C. L. Markert and R. M. Petters, 'Manufactured Hexaparental Mice Show That Adults Are Derived from Three Embryonic Cells' in *Science*, **202** (6 Oct. 1978) 58.

26. K. Moore, *op. cit.* p. 6.

27. *Dorland's Illustrated Medical Dictionary*, 26th edn, Philadelphia: W. B. Saunders Company, 1981. *s.v.*

28. *Ibid.*

Chapter 5

1. Cf. J. M. W. Slack, *From Egg to Embryo*, Cambridge University Press, 1983, pp. 21, 152, Tables 7.1 and 7.3, and pp. 166 and 169; Bruce Alberts *et al.*, *Molecular Biology of the Cell*, New York: Garland Publishing, Inc., 1983, p. 829.

2. Cf. R. G. Edwards, *Conception in the Human Female*, London: Academic Press, 1980, pp. 931–3. A. McLaren 'The Embryo' in *Embryonic and Fetal Development*, Book 2, *Reproduction in Mammals*, eds. C. R. Austin & R. V. Short, Cambridge University Press, 1982, p. 19.; M. B. Renfree, 'Implantation and Placentation' in *Embryonic and Fetal* Development, *ibid.* p. 68, Fig. 2.29.

3. Cf. R. Edwards, *op. cit.* pp. 931–2, where he puts the proportion of monozygotic monoamniotic twins at 1 in 8000 births. Cf. J. Slack, *op cit.* p. 151, who suggests 1 % of identical twins form at the primitive streak stage. Cf. also M. Renfree, *art. cit.* Fig. 2.29 and p. 68.

4. Cf. A. McLaren, *art. cit.* p. 19. Fraternal twinning varies more from country to country with the number per 1000 births being as follows: Japan 2.7; India 6.8; U.S.A. 7.1; Sweden 8.6; England and Wales 8.8; Congo 19.0 and Nigeria 42.0. Cf. ibid. p. 19.

5. Cf. J. Slack, *op. cit*, pp. 165–7 and Table 7.1.

6. P. Parisi, *et al.*, 'Familial Incidence of Twinning' in *Nature*, **304** (1983) 626–8.

7. Cf. R. G. Edwards, *op. cit.* pp. 677 and 733.

8. Cf. L. Mohr and A. Trounson, 'In Vitro Fertilization and Embryo Transfer' in *Clinical In Vitro Fertilization*, eds. C. Wood and A. Trounson, Berlin: Springer Verlag, 1984, pp. 108 and 110. A. Lopata, D. Kohlman and I. Johnson, in 'The Fine Structure of Normal and Abnormal Human Embryos Developed in Culture' in *Fertilization of Human Eggs in Vitro: Biological Basis and Clinical Application*, eds. H. M. Beier and H. R. Linder, Berlin: Springer-Verlag, N. Y.: 1983, pp. 205–7. A. McLaren *art. cit.* p. 5.

9. Cf. Clifford Grobstein, 'The Moral Use of Spare Embryos' in *The Hastings*

Center Report, June, 1982, pp. 5–6: '... up to the eight-cell stage, despite the establishment of *genetic* individuality at fertilization, a multicellular individual is still not present. Since persons, as usually defined, are multicellular individuals, it is difficult to maintain scientifically that a person has come into existence prior to the eight-cell stage.' He goes even further and concludes on account of the possibility of twinning up to two weeks after fertilization: 'the entire pre-implantation period can be regarded scientifically as one of pre-individuality in a developmental sense'. *Ibid.* p. 6.

10. Cf. A. McLaren, *art. cit.* p. 22–3, Table 1.3.
11. Cf. B. Alberts *et al.*, *op. cit.* p. 829. Prior to implantation the embryo loses dry weight since much of the material for its metabolic activity must be found within the embryo. Cf. J. M. W. Slack, *op. cit.* p. 139.
12. I have drawn mainly from the following sources for general information on experimental manipulations of chimaeric embryos: R. L. Gardner, 'Manipulation of Development' in *Embryonic and Fetal Development*, Book 2, *Reproduction in Mammals*, eds. C. R. Austin & R. V. Short, pp. 159–61; A. McLaren, *art. cit.* pp. 9–10; R. G. Edwards, *op. cit.* pp. 732–6.
13. Cf. S. M. Willadsen and C. B. Fehilly, 'The Developmental Potential and Regulatory Capacity of Blastomeres from Two-, Four-, and Eight-Cell Sheep Embryos' in *Fertilization of Human Eggs in Vitro: Biological Basis and Clinical Application*, eds. H. M. Beier and H. R. Linder, Berlin: Springer-Verlag, N.Y.: 1983, pp. 353–7. Cf. Similar work by Willadsen in 'The Developmental Capacity of Blastomeres from 4- and 8-cell Sheep Embryos' in *Journal of Embryology and Experimental Morphology* **65** (1981) 165–72. See also an updated account of this area by C. B. Fehilly and S. M. Willadsen, 'Embryo Manipulation in Farm Animals' in *Oxford Reviews of Reproductive Biology*, ed. J. R. Clarke, Oxford: Clarendon Press, 1986, Vol. 8, pp. 379–413.
14. Cf. C. B. Fehilly and S. M. Willadsen, 'Embryo Manipulation in Farm Animals', *art. cit.* pp. 391–2; C. L. Markert and R. M. Petters, 'Manufactured Hexaparental Mice Show That Adults Are Derived from Three Embryonic Cells' in *Science*, N.Y., **202** (1978) 56–58; C. B. Fehilly, S. M. Willadsen and E. M. Tucker, 'Experimental Chimaerism in Sheep' in *Journal of Reproductive Fertility*, **70** (1984) 347–51.
15. Cf. C. B. Fehilly and S. M. Willadsen, '*Embryo Manipulation in Farm Animals*', *art. cit.* p. 395.
16. *Ibid.* pp. 396–8.
17. Cf. *Ibid.* pp. 402–4.
18. Cf. *ibid.* p. 380; A. McLaren, 'Prelude to Embryogenesis' in *Human Embryo Research: Yes or No?* The Ciba Foundation London: Tavistock Publications, 1986, pp. 6, 10.
19. Cf. A. McLaren, 'The Embryo' in *Embryonic and Fetal Development, Reproduction in Mammals* Bk 2, eds. C. R. Austin & R. V. Short, Cambridge University Press, 1982, p. 3.
20. *Cf.* A. McLaren, *Ibid.* p. 3.
21. Cf. the following sources for information on compaction: A. Lopata *et al.* 'The Fine Structure of Normal and Abnormal Human Embryos Developed in Culture' in *Fertilization of Human Eggs in Vitro: Biological Basis and Clinical Application*, eds. H. M. Beier & H. R. Linder, Berlin: Springer-Verlag, N.Y.: 1983, pp. 190; 205–7; A. McLaren, 'The Embryo', *art. cit.* p. 3.; A. McLaren, 'Prelude to Embryogenesis', *art. cit.* p. 9; R. G. Edwards, *op. cit.* pp. 677–9, 687; 705; 738–9; L. Mohr and A. Trounson *art. cit.* p. 108.
22. The detailed information given here was taken from: A. McLaren, 'Prelude to

embryogenesis' *art. cit.* p. 9; J. M. W. Slack, *op. cit.* pp. 20, 26–7, 139, 144–8; M. A. H. Surani and S. C. Barton, 'Spatial Distribution of Blastomeres is Dependent on Cell Division Order and Interactions in Mouse Morulae' in *Developmental Biology*, **102** (1984) 335–43 and Bruce Alberts *et al., op. cit.* pp. 682–8.

23. *Cf.* R. L. Gardner, 'Origin and Differentiation of Extra-embryonic Tissues in the Mouse' in *International Review of Experimental Pathology*, Vol. 24, N.Y., Academic Press, 1983, pp. 68–71.

24. Cf. M. A. H. Surani and S. C. Barton, *art. cit.* pp. 335–43.

25. Cf. *Ibid.* p. 341.

26. Cf. C. R. Austin, 'The Egg' in *Germ Cells and Fertilization*, Book 1, *Reproduction in Mammals*, eds. C. R. Austin & R. V. Short, Cambridge University Press, 1982, pp. 59–61, where, among other things, he provides a scheme to show the possible routes for parthenogenetic development; A. McLaren, 'The Embryo', *art. cit.*, p. 7; also A. McLaren, 'Reproductive Options, Present and Future' in *Manipulating Reproduction, Reproduction in Mammals*, Bk 5, eds. C. R. Austin & R. V. Short, Cambridge University Press, 1986, p. 189.

27. Cf. J. McGrath and D. Solter, 'Completion of Mouse Embryogenesis Requires Both the Maternal and Paternal Genomes' in *Cell*, **37** (1984) 179–83. Similar conclusions are reported by J. R. Mann & R. H. Lovell-Badge in 'Inviability of parthenogenones is determined by pronuclei, not egg cytoplasm', in *Nature*, **310** (1984) 66–7.

28. Cf. M. A. H. Surani, W. Reik, M. L. Norris and S. C. Barton, 'Influence of germline modifications of homologous chromosomes on mouse development' in *Journal of Embryology and Experimental Morphology*, **97** *Supplement*, 1986, pp. 123–36. See also M. A. H. Surani, S. C. Barton and M. L. Morris 'Development of mouse eggs suggests imprinting of the genome during gametogenesis', in *Nature*, **308** (1984) 548–550; see also the work by the same authors, 'Influence of parental chromosomes on spatial specificity in androgenetic ↔ parthenogenetic chimaeras in the mouse', *Nature*, **326** (1987) 395–7.

29. Cf. K. Moore, *The Developing Human: Clinically Oriented Embryology*, 3rd ed. Philadelphia: W. B. Saunders, 1982, pp. 32–3. IVF researchers suspect they may have had some cases of parthenogenetic development of human eggs when the haploid ovum developed or only one pronucleus appeared. Cf. I. L. Pike in 'Biological Risks of In Vitro Fertilization and Embryo Transfer' in *Clinical In Vitro Fertilization*, eds. C. Wood & A. Trounson, Berlin: Springer-Verlag, 1984, pp. 139 and 143.

30. Cf. R. R. Angell, R. J. Aitken, P. F. A. Van Look, M. A. Lumsden, A. A. Templeton, 'Chromosome Abnormalities in Human Embryos after in Vitro Fertilization' in *Nature* 303 (1983) 336–8.

31. Cf. the following sources used for this section: K. Moore, *op. cit.* pp. 33–69; A. McLaren, 'The Embryo', *art. cit.* 1–25; R. G. Edwards, *op. cit.* pp. 677–88; 705; 724; 732–9; L. Mohr and A. Trounson, *art. cit.* in *Clinical In Vitro Fertilization*, eds. C. Wood & A. Trounson, Berlin: Springer-Verlag, pp. 108–13.

32. Cf. S. B. Fishel *et al.* in 'In Vitro Fertilization of Human Oocytes: Factors Associated with Embryonic Development in Vitro, Replacement of Embryos and Pregnancy' in *Fertilization of Human Eggs in Vitro: Biological Basis and Clinical Application*, eds. H. M. Beier & H. R. Linder, Berlin: Springer-Verlag, N.Y.: 1983, pp. 251–5; Cf. *ibid.*, 'Growth and Differentiation of Rabbit Blastocysts in Defined Culture Media', by H. M. Beier *et al.* pp. 371, 373 and 376.

33. Cf. K. Moore, *op. cit.* pp. 46, 51. Cf. also McLaren, 'The Embryo', *art cit.* p. 22.

34. Cf. A. McLaren. *Ibid.* p. 22, Tab. 1.3 H. M. Beier *et al., art. cit.* p. 371.
35. Cf. R. G. Edwards, *op. cit.*, p. 688; also L. Mohr and A. Trounson, *art cit.*, p. 108.
36. Cf. R. G. Edwards, *op. cit.* pp. 682–3. A. McLaren, 'The Embryo', *art. cit.* pp. 3–4. Edwards elsewhere has something interesting to say about the developing embryo: 'it becomes magnificently organized, switching on its own biochemistry, increasing in size, and preparing itself quickly for implantation in the womb. After that its organs form – the cells gradually become capable of development into heart, lung, brain, eye. What a unique and wonderful process it is, as the increasing number of cells diverge and specialize in a delicate, integrated and coordinated manner.' See 'Four Beautiful Human Blastocysts' in *A Matter of Life*, R. G. Edwards and P. Steptoe, London: Sphere, 1981, p. 91.
37. It is thought that the 'clock' functions chronologically, not dependent on the number of cleavage divisions. On the other hand it could be some sort of 'nuclear memory' that counts mitotic divisions even if cleavage does not follow. Though the timing is more precise in early development, it continues through childhood for the growth of teeth, biological changes at puberty, adulthood etc. right through to old age. Cf. R. G. Edwards, *op. cit.* pp. 682–3; also A. McLaren, 'The Embryo' *art. cit.*, pp. 3–4.
38. Cf. J. Lejeune, 'Biologie, Conscience et Foi' in *Revista di Biologia*, **76**, N. 3, (1983) 463–79 at p. 470.
39. G. C. Liggins, 'The Fetus and Birth', in *Embryonic and Fetal Development, Reproduction in Mammals* Bk 2, eds. C. R. Austin & R. V. Short, Cambridge University Press, 1982, p. 118.
40. Cf. McLaren, 'The Embryo' *art. cit.* p. 4.
41. Cf. *ibid.* p. 3; K. Moore, *op. cit.* pp. 33; 40–42; R. G. Edwards *op. cit.* pp. 684, 736. R. L. Gardner, 'Manipulation of Development', in *Embryonic and Fetal Development, Reproduction in Mammals* Bk 2, eds. C. R. Austin & R. V. Short, Cambridge University Press, 1982, pp. 167–8.
42. Cf. Edwards, *op. cit.* p. 684.
43. Cf. B. Towers, 'Life Before Birth: Human Embryology and the Law of Complexity – Consciousness' in *The Month*, **38** (1967) 34–44, at p. 47.
44. Cf. P. J. O'Mahony and M. Potts, in 'Abortion and the Soul' in *The Month*, **38** (1967) pp. 45–50, at p. 48.
45. Cf. R. G. Edwards *op. cit.* pp. 682–5; 735–9; A. McLaren, 'The Embryo' *art. cit.* pp. 3–4; R. L. Gardner, 'Manipulation of Development', *art. cit.*, pp. 161–3, 167; L. Mohr *et al.* 'Evaluation of Normal and Abnormal Human Embryo Development During Procedures in Vitro' in *Fertilization of Human Eggs in Vitro: Biological Basis and Clinical Application*, eds. H. M. Beier & H. R. Linder, Berlin: Springer-Verlag, 1983, p. 216; H. M. Beier *et al*, 'Growth Differentiation of Rabbit Blastocysts in Defined Culture Media', *ibid.* p. 373; J. M. W. Slack, *op. cit.* pp. 147–8.
46. Cf. R. L. Gardner, 'Manipulation of Development', *art. cit.* pp. 163–7. Cf. C. B. Fehilly and S. M. Willadsen, 'Embryo Manipulation in Farm Animals' in *Oxford Reviews of Reproductive Biology*, Vol. 8, ed. J. R. Clarke, Oxford: Clarendon Press, 1986, p. 398.
47. Cf. R. L. Gardner, 'Manipulation of Development', *art. cit.* pp. 164; 167–8.
48. *Ibid.* p. 168. Cf. also Edwards, *op. cit.* pp. 735–6.
49. Cf. K. Moore, *op. cit.* pp. 45–6; 51; 55–6; 58–9.
50. Cf. R. L. Gardner, 'Manipulation of Development', *art. cit.* p. 168.

Chapter 6

1. Cf. J. M. W. Slack, *From Egg to Embryo: Determinative Events in Early Development*, Cambridge University Press, 1983, pp. 136, 144, 151.
2. Cf. *Ibid.* pp. 32–4.
3. Cf. *Ibid.* pp. 3–8; 151–2.
4. Cf. *Ibid.* p. 152.
5. *Cf. Ibid.* pp. 44–5.
6. I have relied on the following for details here: K. Moore, *The Developing Human: Clinically Oriented Embryology*, Philadelphia: W. B. Saunders, 1982, pp. 53–5; also R. L. Gardner, 'Manipulation of Development' in *Embryonic and Fetal Development, Reproduction in Mammals*, Bk 2, Cambridge University Press, 1982, pp. 167–8.
7. Cf., K. Moore, *op. cit.* pp. 60–5.
8. Cf. A. McLaren, in 'Prelude to Embryogenesis' in *Human Embryo Research: Yes or No?*, The Ciba Foundation, London: Tavistock Publications, 1986, pp. 11–12. Much of this paragraph is taken from this chapter of McLaren. Cf. also L. W. Browder, *Developmental Biology*, Philadelphia: Saunders, 1984, pp. 609–15, where he describes the appearance of the primitive streak for a chick, pointing out the great similarities found in the human in this respect.
9. Cf. R. L. Gardner, 'Manipulation of Development', *art. cit.* pp. 167–8; Cf. M. H. L. Snow, 'Techniques for Separating Early Embryonic Tissues' in *Methods in Mammalian Reproduction*, ed. J. C. Daniel Jr, London: Academic Press, N.Y., 1978, p. 169.
10. Cf. R. G. Edwards, *Conception in the Human Female*, London: Academic Press, 1980, pp. 931–2; A. McLaren, 'The Embryo', in *Embryonic and Fetal Development, Reproduction in Mammals*, Bk 2, eds. C. R. Austin and R. V. Short, Cambridge University Press, 1982, p. 19; M. B. Renfree, *Ibid.* 'Implantation and Placentation', p. 67; For an interesting discussion on the individuality of twins, Cf. S. J. Gould, 'Living with Connections: Are Siamese Twins One Person or Two' in *Natural History*, **91** (Nov. 1982) 18–22.
11. K. Moore, *op. cit.* p. 54.
12. Cf. 'Where to Draw the Line?', in *Proceedings of the Royal Institution*, G. B. **56** (1984) 101–21. By courtesy of the Director of the Royal Institution.
13. Cf. A. McLaren, 'Prelude to Embryogenesis', *art. cit.* p. 22.
14. Cf. *Ibid.* p. 14 where Anne McLaren expresses the same thought in regard to the formation of the individual mouse embryo proper: '... the 'embryo' as a continuous entity could be traced back from birth only as far as the primitive streak stage (six days after fertilization in mice), and that the 'embryo' that develops from fertilization onwards is a different entity, which includes and gives rise to the 'embryo' that grows into a fetus and neonate but is in no way coextensive with it.' I think a parallel can be drawn from the development of the larva and pupa into a fruit fly. The pupa has been compared to a walking and feeding counterpart of the mammalian extraembryonic membranes, designed to carry and nourish the imaginal cells that will give origin to the adult body. Cf. *Molecular Biology of the Cell*, ed. Bruce Alberts *et al.* New York: Garland Publishing, Inc. 1983, pp. 836–8.
15. Cf. A. McLaren, 'Prelude to Embryogenesis', *art. cit.* pp. 7 and 12. Cf. also K. Moore, *op. cit.* pp. 53–91.
16. J. J. Diamond, M.D., 'Abortion, Animation and Homonization' in *Theological Studies*, **36** (1975) 315.

17. J. Mahoney, S.J., *Bioethics and Belief*, London: Sheed and Ward, 1984, pp. 66–7.

18. Quoted in *The Morality of Abortion: Legal and Historical Perspectives*, ed. John T. Noonan, Jr, Harvard, Mass: Harvard Univ. Press, 1970, p. 66.

19. *Report of the Committee of Inquiry into Human Fertilisation and Embryology*, Chairman, Baroness Mary Warnock, Department of Social Security, London; Her Majesty's Stationery Office, 1984, p. 66.

20. *Ibid.* p. 65.

21. *Ibid.* p. 59. The *Warnock Report* has an excellent summary of early human development on pp. 58–60. It agrees with K. Moore's account in practically every detail.

22. *Ibid.* p. 66.

23. *The Committee to Consider the Social, Ethical and Legal Issues Arising from In Vitro Fertilization: Report on the Disposition of Embryos Produced by In Vitro Fertilization*, Melbourne, August, 1984.

24. *Ibid.* pp. 27, 46.

25. *Ibid.* p. 32. Confirmation of the Report's use of the term 'entity' in a non-technical and broad sense is had in Rev. Dr Francis Harman's Statement of Dissent in Appendix A: 'In the context of the Committee's discussions, by the term 'embryo' is understood the entity deriving from the fusion (whether intra-uterine or extra-uterine) of human sperm and ovum throughout that phase of its existence which runs from the moment of fusion up until the moment of delivery or of death if unfortunately that should precede delivery.' pp. 62–3. The Committee took the ordinary meaning of 'embryo' in human language and referred to it equivalently as an 'individual and genetically unique human entity' without specifying the type of unity that remained in the embryo after the fertilized egg began to divide and multiply cells. In ordinary language we refer to a watch in the singular as an entity or thing, without thereby denying that *it* is really made up of many parts that actually have their own separate existence.

26. *Ibid.* p. 47.

27. Cf. *Ibid.* p. 47; *Warnock Report*, p. 66. The *Waller Report* also refers to the same limit for experimentation on human embryos recommended by the Medical Research Council of Great Britain, (MRC) 1982, (p. 42) and the National Health and Medical Research Council (N.H. & M.R.C.) of Australia, p. 41. The same limit of 14 days after fertilization is placed by the Ethics Advisory Board of the U.S.A. Dept. of Health in its Report on IVF. Cf. P. Singer and D. Wells, *The Reproduction Revolution: New Ways of Making Babies*, Oxford: Oxford University Press, 1984, p. 210.

The *Warnock Report*, *op. cit.* p. 65 indicated that the British Medical Association (Cf. *British Medical Journal*, **286** (1984) 1594–5.) likewise favoured a 14 day limit on experimentation, whilst the Royal College of Physicians suggested the end of implantation which is about day 12 or 13. In its Report the Ethics Committee of the Royal College of Obstetricians and Gynaecologists suggested a 17 day limit as early neural development began then (March 1983). Perhaps they were concerned about the possibility of pain being experienced from about that time on. Again it could be that some development of the nervous system was considered necessary for a person to actually exist.

28. Cf. Mary Warnock, 'Do Human Cells Have Rights?' in *Bioethics*, **I** (1987) 11–12.

29. *Human Embryo Experimentation in Australia: Senate Select Committee on the*

Human Embryo Experimentation Bill 1985, Canberra: Australian Government Publishing Service, 1986, p. 25, 3.7.

30. Cf. A. McLaren, 'Prelude to Embryogenesis' *art. cit.* p. 12; K. Moore, *op. cit.* p. 33.

31. *Human Embryo Experimentation in Australia, op. cit.* p. 29, 3.21.

32. Cf. 'Pregnancy Losses and Birth Defects' in *Embryonic and Fetal Development, Reproduction in Mammals*, Bk 2, eds. C. R. Austin & R. V. Short, Cambridge University Press, 1982, pp. 146–7.

33. Cf. K. Moore, *op. cit.* pp. 36, 49 presents a range of estimates from various authorities; Cf. J. D. Biggers 'In Vitro Fertilization and Embryo Transfer in Human Beings' in *The New England Journal of Medicine*, Feb. 1981, pp. 336–42. He concludes that only 31% of human eggs exposed to sperm are born alive; Cf. R. V. Short for similar results in 'When a Conception Fails to Become a Pregnancy' in *Symposium on Maternal Recognition of Pregnancy, Excerpta Medica*, London, 1978, pp. 377–87; Cf. also J. F. Miller *et al.* in 'Fetal Loss After Implantation: A Prospective Study' in *The Lancet*, Sept. 13, 1980, pp. 554–6. They found a maximum conception rate of 36%; Cf. T. W. Hilgers who argues for a loss rate of less than 15% in 'Human Reproduction: Three Issues for the Moral Theologian' in *Theological Studies*, **38** (1977) 147–9. A trial of natural family planning with 209 women showed no spontaneous abortions after a positive HCG test; Cf. 'A Randomized Prospective Study of the Use-effectiveness of Two Methods of Natural Family Planning', M. Wade *et al.* in *American Journal of Obstetrics and Gynaecology*, Oct. 1981, pp. 368–76.

34. Cf. Ashley and O'Rourke *op. cit. Health Care Ethics: A Theological Analysis*, St Louis: The Catholic Health Association of the USA, 1982, p. 223.

35. Cf. P. Jacobs, 'Pregnancy Losses and Birth Defects', *art. cit.* p. 147. She puts it at 25%. Dame Josephine Barnes puts it slightly less: '*Spontaneous abortion* of an intrauterine pregnancy is common and occurs in at least 20 per cent of all pregnancies.' Cf. 'abortion' title in *Dictionary of Medical Ethics*, eds. A. S. Duncan, G. R. Dunstan and R. B. Welbourn, Darton, Longman & Todd, London, 1981, p. 1.

36. Cf. 'The Beginning of Human Life' by Rev. Dr. T. J. Connolly, in *Faith and Culture: Contemporary Questions*, Catholic Institute of Sydney, Manly, 1983, p. 96.

37. Cf. Anne McLaren, 'Reproductive Options, Present and Future', in *Manipulating Reproduction*, Book 5, *Reproduction in Mammals* eds. C. R. Austin & R. V. Short, Cambridge University Press, 1986, pp. 178–80. A note on p. 178 refers to the use of 'proembryo' in *Henderson's Dictionary of Biological Terms*, 1979. Cf. also Anne McLaren, 'Prelude to Embryogenesis', *art. cit.* p. 12; Anne McLaren, 'Why study early human development?', in *New Scientist*, 24 April 1986, p. 49.

GLOSSARY

accidental form: an intrinsic principle of being that affects the way something exists without changing the kind of being that it is. Examples are size, shape and qualities that admit degrees of change, e.g. temperature, colour etc.

amnion: Extraembryonic membrane, that lines the chorion and encloses the embryo–fetus in the so-called amniotic fluid.

blastocyst: a hollow ball of cells, filled with fluid, that forms about four days after fertilization and prior to the beginning of the process of implantation.

blastomeres: the daughter cells that derive from the first and subsequent cleavages of the zygote.

chimaera: an organism formed by the aggregation of cells taken from different genotypes. Chimaeric embryos may occur naturally or artificially.

chorion: outermost cellular extraembryonic membrane.

chorionic villi: finger-like projections growing from the external surface of the chorion that contribute to the formation of the placenta.

chromosomes: Linear threads of DNA that transmit genetic information through genes spaced along their entire length. In the human somatic cell there are normally two sets of 23 chromosomes including the two (XX or XY) that determine the sex of the individual. Each gamete normally contains only one set of 23 chromosomes.

cleavage (mitosis): The process whereby the cells divide and thereby multiply to become similar identical daughter cells during early embryo development.

conceptus: this term refers to the products of fertilization. It includes the embryo proper as well as extraembryonic structures and tissues that develop from the zygote (e.g. placenta).

codon: a series of three adjacent bases in one polynucleotide chain of a DNA or RNA molecule which codes for a specific amino acid during the synthesis of proteins.

diploid: having two sets of chromosomes, usually one paternal and one maternal; twice the haploid number (in humans 46).

DNA: deoxyribonucleic acid, the primary constituent of chromosomes and the basis of the genetic code and inherited traits.

embryo: early or preimplantation embryo refers to the first two weeks after the formation of the zygote. Embryo technically refers to the stage from the third to eighth week of development. Often the term embryo also encompasses development from the beginning up to the eighth week.

entity: a thing that really exists and cannot be reduced to being simply the object of some conscious activity. Broadly speaking, the term may refer to anything that is real, even relationships between persons or things (e.g. bank, corporation, Church); strictly speaking it refers to something real that exists independently in its own right as one being (e.g. molecule, cat or even God.)

epiblast: also called primitive, or primary embryonic ectoderm. The non-endodermal part of the inner cell mass of the blastocyst. From it are derived during the third week all three germ layers of the entire embryo proper (ectoderm, mesoderm and endoderm). Hence this tissue is multipotential.

fertilization: process that begins when a sperm contacts the plasma membrane of an egg and is completed with the formation of a zygote at syngamy.

fetus: the developing human individual from the ninth week after fertilization until birth.

gamete: a mature reproductive cell, usually haploid, e.g. sperm or ovum.

gastrula: the name given to the embryo during gastrulation when the bilaminar embryonic disc becomes a trilaminar embryonic disc from days 14 to 19.

gene: the basic unit of inheritance, comprising a specific sequence of nucleotides on a DNA chain, that has a specific function and occupies a specific place on a chromosome.

genome: the complete set of hereditary factors, as contained in the haploid assortment of chromosomes. Frequently used broadly to refer to the complete genetic material for any cell or organism.

genotype: the hereditary or genetic constitution of an individual or of a cell, usually referring only to the nuclear material.

haploid: having one set of chromosomes as normally carried by a gamete (23 in humans).

hydatidiform mole: a placental abnormality composed of grape-like clusters of chorionic villi. It is the product of an abnormal fertilization where live placental tissue is formed without any embryo.

hylomorphism: referring to the metaphysical theory that explains the unity and constitution of bodies in terms of the co-principles of matter and form.

inner cell mass (ICM): the cluster of cells within the blastocyst closely adhering together on the trophectoderm. They derive from the cells in the centre of the morula. The embryo proper develops from some of these cells.

meiosis: division of a diploid nucleus into four nuclei, each with half the number of the chromosomes of the parent nucleus and with a mix of both maternal and paternal chromosome sets, resulting in both sperm and egg with 23 genetically unique chromosomes each.

metaphysics: the branch of philosophy that explains reality in terms of concepts, causes and first principles that are not restricted to what is given in experience (empirical).

mitosis: process of diploid cell division where the chromosomes double and then separate longitudinally and normally give origin to two identical diploid daughter cells, each with a complete set of pairs of chromosomes.

morula (the Latin for mulberry): once the proliferating cells from the fertilized egg compact, they appear at the 12–16-cell stage like a mulberry. Hence the name is applied about three days after fertilization.

ontological: refers to actual existence in reality as distinct from in thought or in the imagination.

ontological individual: a single concrete entity that exists as a distinct being and is not an aggregation of smaller things nor merely a part of a greater whole; hence its unity is said to be intrinsic. A single member of a class of beings or species but not a group.

oocyte: the immature female germ cell. It is called an *ovum* when it matures after the penetration of the sperm during fertilization and the completion of the second meiotic division.

primary endoderm, also called *endoderm* and *hypoblast*: the layer of cells that forms under the inner cell mass facing the blastocyst cavity.

prime matter: a real potential principle of being, which together with the actuating influence of the form, constitutes a body.

primitive streak: a piling up of cells on the caudal end of the embryonic disc, providing the earliest evidence of the embryonic axis and the formation of the embryo proper.

primordium: the earliest sign or stage of development of an organ or other structure.

proembryo: the developing cells produced by the division of the zygote before the formation of the embryo proper at the appearance of the primitive streak. Also called pre-embryo.

pronucleus: the egg or sperm nucleus after penetration of the egg by the sperm.

RNA: ribonucleic acid, which is found in the cytoplasm of the cell and directs protein synthesis. Messenger RNA (mRNA) transfers the genetic information from the DNA to the ribosomes that are the protein forming system of the cell.

substantial form: an intrinsic actuating principle of being that makes prime matter be a specific kind of bodily being. Also called soul on life-principle for living bodies: vegetative soul for plants, sensitive soul for animals. In humans it is simply called soul (spiritual) but it functions as the substantial form.

syngamy: the mingling of the male and female haploid chromosome sets following the breakdown of the pronuclear membranes. This results in the formation of the zygote.

teratoma: a new and uncontrolled growth of cells and tissues that are the product of an abnormal fertilization without any potential to develop into an embryo proper or fetus.

totipotency: this represents the capacity (potential) of a cell or a cluster of cells to produce the whole (total) embryo and fetus with all its extraembryonic membranes and tissues. Pluripotency or multipotency is similar but is restricted to represent the capacity to produce a variety of parts and tissues but not the whole embryo and fetus.

trophectoderm: the cells that form the outer wall of the blastocyst.

trophoblast: the layer of cells derived from the outer trophectoderm layer of the blastocyst. It attaches the blastocyst to the uterine wall.

zona pellucida: a thick, transparent noncellular layer of uniform thickness surrounding the oocyte, zygote and early embryo for several days, when it degenerates and allows the embryo to emerge or hatch out.

zygote: the fertilized egg; the single cell that is formed when the two haploid sets of chromosomes in the pronuclei of the male and female gametes come together at syngamy. Also used loosely to refer to the early embryo during the first few weeks.

INDEX

The index includes subjects and names appearing directly in the text. The *Glossary* should be consulted for meanings of scientific and philosophical terms. The bibliographical references in the *Notes* give the names of all authors consulted.